Yoga for Everyone!
Chair Yoga
Hatha Yoga
Gentle Yoga

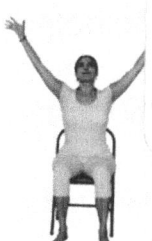 

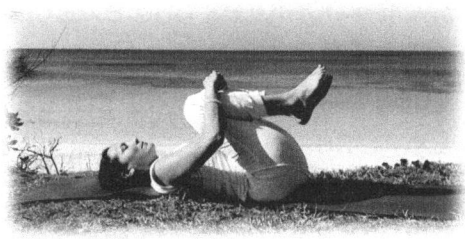

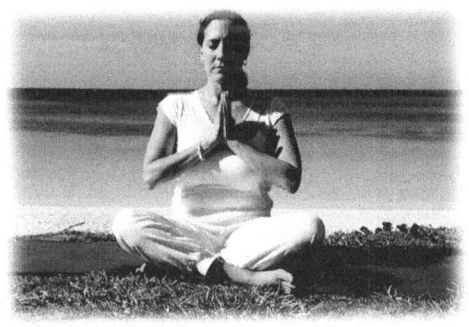

SunLight Chair Yoga: yoga for everyone!

Copyright © 2018 Stacie Dooreck

Not all of the yoga postures and exercises in this book are suitable for everyone. Consult your physician or medical provider for concerns prior to doing these exercises. The instructions and suggestions in this book are in no way intended as a substitute for medical counseling.

SunLight Yoga Publishers
www.sunlightyoga.com

ISBN-13: 978-0-9916250-3-1
Health & Fitness / Yoga
Printed in the United States of America

DEDICATION

To my father who brought yoga into my life and continues to keep it in his.

To my mom, who supported our vegetarian diet.

To the yogis of past and present, who share these teachings to better humanity, the earth and ourselves.

ACKNOWLEDGMENTS

To all of my yoga students, who were also my teachers, keeping me inspired to learn more ways to adapt and share yoga.

To all yoga masters including Swami Sivananda, Krishnamacharya, Swami Vishnu Devananda, Swami Sachidnananda, BKS Iyengar, Yogi Bhajan, Dharma Mittra and Lilias Folan. Their teachings are timeless yet perfect for the modern age.

I am beyond grateful to the lineages of yoga that I have learned from, including Sivananda Yoga for the foundation of Hatha Yoga (*asanas*, *pranayama*, relaxation and meditation), Integral Gentle Yoga and Kundalini Yoga.

FOREWARD

I never intended to be an author. After many years of teaching and practicing yoga, I simply wanted to share the teachings with more people. I wanted to show how they could be adapted, to be of benefit to all. I was teaching and practicing yoga many years before I got Lyme disease, a chronic illness that lasted through much of my 20s and 30s. I learned how to adapt yoga then, not only for my students, but for my own needs.

My first two books on Chair Yoga included seated and standing yoga postures, using a chair for support. This book offers more ideas, including the *Hatha Yoga asana* (posture) with several ways to adapt it. This includes adapting it for a more gentle practice, called "Gentle Yoga', as well as the Chair Yoga versions of the posture. This book shows some of the many ways to adapt yoga. The possibilities are endless so that everyone can practice yoga at all stages of life. Yoga truly is for everyone!

In this book, only some of the benefits are listed for each pose and yoga practice. These are suggested benefits, based on my own experiences. Try it for yourself and see how the practice will benefit you.

DISCLAIMER

By performing any yoga or exercises in this book, you are performing them at your own risk. Stacie Dooreck, SunLight Yoga, www.sunlightyoga.com will not be responsible or liable for any injury or harm you sustain as a result of this yoga video, nor for information shared on our website or in related videos.

Please consult with your medical professional before starting a yoga practice or any exercise routine, to find out your specific precautions and modifications needed, based on your medical condition. This book notes some general precautions, but does not include all modifications or precautions for all injuries and conditions. Not all of the yoga postures and exercises in this book are suitable for everyone. Consult your physician or medical provider for concerns prior to doing these exercises. Yoga heals and helps when it is practiced in a safe way that does not create pain or discomfort. Yoga is for everyone but we are all unique.

QUOTES FROM THE MASTERS

"Expand. Evolve. Grow. Forget not the goal. Awake. Achieve the goal." Swami Sivananda

"Yoga is the journey of the self, through the self, to the self." The Bhagavad Gita

"Health is wealth. Peace of mind is happiness. Yoga shows the way." Swami Vishnudevananda

"If you can breathe, you can do yoga." Krishnamacharya

"The Nature of the Absolute is Peace: Absolute Peace, Perfect Peace, Unutterable Peace." Swami Sivananda

"Serve, love, give, purify, meditate, realize. Be good, do good, be kind, be compassionate. Inquire 'who am I' know the Self and be free. Concentrate, meditate, attain Self-realization." –Swami Sivananda

"When I wake up in the morning, I know that it's going to be the best day of my life. I never think about what I can't do. Make sure positive thoughts are the first ones you think in the morning. And never procrastinate." Tao Porchon Lynch, -100 year old yoga teacher

Table of Contents

Yoga for Everyone!

Yoga for Everyone!

1

In Chapter 1, Yoga for Everyone!

- Introduction

- What is yoga?

- The five points of yoga

- The four paths of yoga?

- Simple ways to practice

- What is Hatha Yoga?

- What is Yoga Asana?

- What is Gentle Yoga?

•How often to practice

There are many ways to practice yoga, including:

- Hatha Yoga
- Gentle Yoga
- Chair Yoga
- Meditation
- Relaxation
- Yogic Diet
- Breathing Exercises
- Positive Thinking
- Karma Yoga

Introduction

After 24 years of practicing and teaching yoga, many of those years I had to adapt the teachings to include Chair Yoga and Gentle Yoga, so that everyone could benefit and practice, regardless of their physical condition. In this book, I wanted to share with you various ways in which you can practice yoga, to make it comfortable, useful and beneficial for your unique condition. We are all unique, so your practice may need to vary as well, according to your needs.

Take a moment to pause and consider this fact: there is only one of each us on this planet with this particular body and mind. What an amazing miracle, to be in this physical body and to know that no one else in the world will experience the body, sensations and emotions in the exact same way as you do. Therefore, you can practice yoga *asanas* (postures) and breathing exercises in different ways, at various stages of our life and even at various times of the day, based on our unique needs. Depending on your current condition of health, mobility and ability, you can always adapt the practice. This may be adapted also at different times the day or only during periods while healing from an injury or an illness.

The adaptions needed may also need to change from day to day.

Yoga is extremely diverse in terms of practices and techniques and gives us many tools to find more balance, strength, flexibility and peace. This includes increasing balance, strength, flexibility and peace, for both the body and the mind. Regardless of your physical condition there is always a way to practice yoga. Yoga is not just the physical postures anyway, as many people think. However, even the postures can be adapted to meet all conditions. Yoga is the most helpful when it is practiced in a safe and beneficial way.

What is yoga?

So what is yoga anyway? Yoga or "union" is an ancient science to help us reach a greater connection with ourselves and the world around us. Yoga includes postures *(asanas)*, breathing exercises *(pranayama)*, chanting, relaxation, meditation, positive thinking, serving humanity and healthy and balanced vegetarian (or vegan) eating and living. Everyone can benefit from yoga. The benefits are numerous ranging from chronic pain relief, improving concentration, balance and quality of sleep, to increasing a sense of general well-being and peace of mind.

When there are physical, energetic, time or other "limitations," the benefits of yoga can still be experienced. When yoga is done in ways that are comfortable, safe and within range of one's current capabilities, the healing, balancing and transformative effects of yoga can occur. Often when we are sick, injured, fatigued or busy at the office, the last thing we think we can do is yoga. But when we modify it to meet our current needs, instead of avoiding the practice altogether, yoga can bring peace of mind, inner and outer strength, flexibility (mental and physical), stress relief, vitality, energy, overall well-being, balance, joy and deep healing. Yoga is for everyone!

The word *yoga* comes from the Sanskrit language, meaning to "yoke" or "join". The "yoking" or "joining" or connecting of the individual self (soul) with the Universal or Cosmic Self (Soul) is yoga. It is the connection of our individual selves to all that exists in the universe, including every human being, animal, tree and atom. On a simple level, yoga connects the body, mind and Spirit, often using the breath as a tool to connect those parts. Yoga also unifies, balances and harmonizes our physical, emotional, mental and spiritual selves.

Yoga is a science of sorts. You must not believe any claims until you try it for yourself and experience its benefits firsthand. The benefits are as infinite as our true selves. With practice, anyone can experience this.

Patanjali, a sage of India consolidated yoga into stages or limbs (*ashtanga* in Sanskrit) known as the 8 limbs of yoga. These include ethics *(yamas)* such as nonviolence or *ahimsa* in Sanskrit, truthfulness *(satya)* and study of the true Self *(svadhyaya)*. After the ethical standards of what to do and not do for living a life with true integrity, Patanjali notes the third limb as yoga *asana* or posture. The yoga postures in this book include showing adaptions using chairs and gentle variations, with and without props, of traditional or more modern variations of yoga postures and exercises.

The Five Points of Yoga

A simple way to think yoga can be summarized as a full lifestyle. Swami Vishnudevananda condensed the essence of the yoga teachings into five principles for physical and mental health and

Yoga for Everyone!

spiritual growth:

- Proper Exercises — *asana*

- Proper Breathing — *pranayama*

- Proper Relaxation — *savasana*

- Proper Diet — vegetarian

- Positive Thinking and Meditation — *dhyana*

Using these five principals for a holistic yogic lifestyle brings inner peace, outer health and harmony with the animals and the earth. Using these principles can contribute more simplicity, more peace and greater harmony to your life.

According to the Yoga Sutras, following the limb of yoga *asana* is *pranayama*, or yogic breathing practices, for balancing and/or increasing the *prana* (vital life force). Then comes *pratyahara*, which is turning the senses inward. After that is *dharana* or concentration and *dhyana* (meditation). This leads to the final stage of *Samadhi*, which is the realization that all is One and is said to be a state of pure ecstasy.

Although these stages can go in the above order, they may also overlap and vary in sequence. You can also practice several of these at once. For example, taking a slow, deep breath during the yoga posture while concentrating deeply can be considered doing an *asana* (yoga posture), *pranayama* (yogic breathing exercises) and *dharana* (concentration) simultaneously. Perhaps you can also ease into a state of *dhyana* (meditation) during the practice. Each time you practice yoga is an opportunity to be present and observe yourself without judgment. And of course, don't forget to enjoy the journey!

Swami Sachidananda explains it as such: "The human body is a temple. Keep it strong and supple. Treat it gently. The codes of living, *Yama* and *Niyama*, are the first two limbs of the eight branches of Yoga. The third is asana--Yoga postures that purify the physical body. Never ignore the body since it is the most important instrument. Whatever you do, you need a body. That's why the ancient Yoga teachings always emphasized taking good care of the body. In almost all the great religious traditions this is indirectly said, but not as openly or with such emphasis as in Yoga. To purify the body we practice the disciplines of Hatha Yoga, which includes the *asanas* or--postures and *pranayama*-- the breathing techniques, which take care of the health of the physical body. This carries over into diet too. Avoid anything that contains toxins or that unnecessarily stimulates your body; try to eliminate alcohol and tobacco. Without purity of the body it's very difficult to purify the mind."

What are the Four Paths of Yoga?

Most people think of yoga as the physical postures only. However there are so many ways to practice yoga. In fact, some of the yoga practices have nothing to do with the exercises or postures at all. There are basically four main paths of Yoga, which are Karma Yoga, Bhakti Yoga, Raja Yoga and Jnana Yoga. Karma Yoga is the path of action, or selfless service. Volunteer work may be a form of Karma Yoga, or any action to serve humanity (or the animals). This includes acting without expectation, meaning you are not performing the action for anything in return. Swami Sivananda said "Man generally plans to get the fruits of his works before he starts any kind of work. The mind is so framed that it cannot think of any kind of work without remuneration or reward. A selfish man cannot do any service. He will weigh the work and the money in a balance. Selfless Service is unknown to him."

Bhakti Yoga is the path of devotion. Some Bhakti Yogis chant the names of the Divine as the main form of practice, to cultivate devotion and love. I myself listen to yoga chants and attend many *kirtans* (call and response chanting) and know firsthand the level of joy and even bliss, this practice can bring. People with an emotional nature may be drawn to this path.

Jnana Yoga is some times called the yoga of wisdom or knowledge. Reading spiritual texts such as the Bhagavad Gita, the Torah or Bible may be considered Jnana Yoga. Those with an intellectual nature may find this path appealing.

Raja Yoga means the "Royal or Kingly Yoga", which practices techniques to control the body, mind and senses, focusing on meditation. As mentioned earlier, the Yoga Sutras of Patanjali, a text of 196 aphorisms, summarized 8 limbs (*ashtanga yoga)*, which includes ethical guidelines or ethical standards, called *yamas* in Sanskrit and self-disciplines called *nimyamas*, as the base for yoga practice. These guidelines include non-violence *(ahimsa)*, truthfulness *(satyam)*, contentment *(santosha)*, non-greediness *or* possessiveness *(aparigraha)* and truthfulness *(satya)*. The remaining limbs are yoga postures *(asanas)*, breathing exercises *(pranayama)*, withdrawal of the senses (*pratyahara*), concentration *(dharana),* meditation *(dhyana)* and ultimate consciousness or final liberation *(samadhi).* Hatha Yoga is apart of Raja Yoga, which is discussed in detail below. This is the branch of Yoga that includes the yoga postures *(asanas).*

What is Hatha Yoga?

In Sanskrit, *ha* means sun and *tha* means moon. Hatha Yoga essentially means 'sun and moon union'. Using the symbols of sun and moon as pairs of opposites, we are basically finding balance when practicing yoga. This is because we are working in such a way, to use the body, mind and breath to restore harmony and equanimity.

When I was in high school I had a neck injury that caused great discomfort. When suggested from a chiropractor to do yoga, I tried a Lilias Folan Yoga video, then on a VHS tape, since this was before the days of seeing yoga studios all over (or DVD players). Within one 30-minute video session my months of prior neck pain, as well as other tensions and anxieties had completely vanished. I was shown right away the incredible benefits of a simple yoga practice and continued to practice for 30 minutes daily after my high school classes.

Although my neck pain had vanished, I felt a deep peace after each practice session so when I was in college I continued to practice daily in my dorm room, memorizing the video sequence I practiced in high school and then using the Sivananda Companion to Yoga book, where I learned my first 1.5 hour sequence. Eventually, because my father was practicing yoga already, by the time I was in college I knew where to go to attend my first class: the Sivananda Yoga Center in NYC. This included the full aspects of *Hatha Yoga*, which started each class with mantras, chanting and breathing techniques to create energy and balance the nervous system.

Yoga ultimately gave me so much more than relief of neck tension, which was my first and only intent to start the practice. Since then it has given me tools to bring more balance, flexibility, strength and peace to my body, mind and emotions and gives me a safe space to focus inside of myself, regardless of what is occurring in my external world. Because of these immense benefits I continued on in my second year of college to live in an ashram for a month and learn to teach yoga.

I now happily share the teachings of yoga with others, so that they too can improve the quality of their lives and health (in both body and mind) and connect to their true innermost Self.

In many large US cities you see so many people doing yoga now and it is even all over the news and media. India had their first International Day of Yoga June 21, 2015. I happened to be visiting India that day and got to practice in the motherland of yoga, where nearby they gathered over 38,000 yogis in Delhi to practice. The Prime Minister of India when presenting the idea of International Yoga Day to the United Nations said that "Yoga should not be just an exercise for us, but it should be a means to get connected with the world and with nature," and also said that yoga is "India's gift." And by December, over 177 countries were involved in this day, including the USA, Iran, France and so many more. I agree completely, yoga is a true gift India brought to this world.

What is Asana?

One of the practices of Hatha Yoga includes yoga *asana*. A yoga *asana* is a posture done in a meditative way. Yoga Sutras 2.46 says in Sanskrit *sthirasukham aasanam*, which means that yoga postures is that which is firm yet relaxed, or translates in another way as "steady and easeful."

Many people know of Sun Salutations, Downward Facing Dog and Headstand Poses, but there are so many more. There is a yogic text from the 17th century, called the Gheranda Samthita, that says there are many postures as species. "All together there are as many *asanas* as there are species of living beings. Shiva has taught 8,400,000. Of these, eighty-four are preeminent, of which thirty-two are useful in the world of mortals."

The Yoga Sutras goes on to say how to master a yoga posture. It says in Sanskrit *prayatna shaithilya ananta samapattibhyam,* which means that the asana (posture) is mastered by releasing tension and meditating on the Infinite or Unlimited." (Yoga Sutra 2.47)

What is Gentle Yoga?

Gentle Yoga is a modern day term that lets the practitioner know the Hatha Yoga *asanas* and breathing techniques are done, simply put as the term suggests, in a 'gentle' way, which may be adapted from the traditional way of practicing. This allows greater healing, support and balance, especially for those with limited mobility, injuries, pre or post surgery or during or after an illness. It also may be useful for those with limited mobility due to age or lack of exercise. If you are new to yoga (at any age), or for those who haven't practiced in a while, a Gentle Yoga class or home session is quite useful. Within a Gentle Yoga class or home practice, some postures can be adapted while others may not need to be. Chair Yoga can be included as well into a Gentle Yoga practice, for only some or all of the yoga *asanas* (postures). See the following chapter to read more about Chair Yoga.

Integrating Yoga Into Our Lives

Using the five principals mentioned before (proper exercises, proper breathing, proper relaxation, proper diet, positive thinking and meditation), for a holistic yogic lifestyle for inner peace, outer health and harmony (with ourselves, the animals and the earth), plus some additional ideas as suggested in the chapter called Yogic Lifestyle, yoga can contribute to a life of more simplicity, peace and greater harmony.

Since yoga is so beneficial, let's not wait

another minute to get to started. The good news is that you can start right you where are, right now, with a simple, slow and deep breath: inhale, then exhale, and repeat.

Yoga Practice

This book includes yoga warm-ups, exercises, postures *(asanas),* breathing practices and simple meditations. It will show options for a Hatha Yoga practice (without a chair or props), a Gentle Yoga adaption of the Hatha Yoga posture when available, and a Chair Yoga option for each yoga pose. Find which one is best for your needs so that the practice is comfortable and easeful. This way the body and mind can relax deeply and receive it's benefits.

This book includes some suggested English affirmations as well. Although traditionally in the yoga posture you simply breathe and focus on the breath, some positive thinking affirmations may be useful too. You can repeat them silently as you breathe and enjoy the posture or on it's own.

How Often to Practice

Consistent daily practice is the best way to see progress, whether to alleviate pain, increase physical strength and flexibility or to feel more at peace mentally and emotionally. If your schedule does not allow a 30 or 60-minute session daily, which would be ideal, you can also create a 5-10 minute session in the morning, and a 10 minute session in the evening. Remembering that Yoga is not just the postures but includes breathing exercises, meditation and also how we eat (see the Yogic Diet chapter), then integrating yoga into our daily lives can happen gradually and easefully.

It is also best to practice daily and consistently, to create a refuge of inner peace and harmony that you can tap into whenever life gets challenging. Often people will practice yoga or meditate when stress levels are high, when health problems arise or there is a crisis. However, if you have an established practice prior, and keep consistent, regardless of outer circumstances, you will be well trained to calm the mind, or heal the body. Although it is beneficial to start or practice yoga at any phase of life, it is most useful when practiced consistently.

"The misery which is not yet come is to be avoided." Yoga Sutras 1.4 (in Sanskrit: *heyan duhkham anagatam*)

Yoga Sutras also says in Sanskrit, *Sah tu dirgha kala nairantaira satkara asevitah dridha bhumih,* which means that when that practice is done for a long time, without a break, and with sincere devotion, then the practice becomes a firmly rooted, stable and solid foundation.

Yoga is a way to integrate the body and mind to feel connected to the breath and Spirit. The practices below can help. So let's begin.

"Anyone who practices can obtain success in yoga but not one who is lazy. Constant practice alone is the secret of success."
Hatha Yoga Pradipika

Chair Yoga

2

Practice yoga:

- At work
- At home
- If injured
- While traveling
- Ore or post surgery
- During an illness
- In a wheelchair

Yoga is for everyone!

What is Chair Yoga?

Chair Yoga is simply yoga done in a chair or wheelchair, (seated or standing), using the chair as a prop for support and stability. The main difference between yoga and chair yoga is that while the yoga postures are sometimes adapted from traditional postures, we are using the chair as support as well. Being creative makes yoga accessible for all.

In this book, my suggested yoga session includes centering, yoga warm-ups, yoga exercises and postures, concentration and breathing exercises, yogic relaxation, meditation and chanting. Although any one of these elements alone can bring great benefit, practicing all of them will give the maximum results for a healthy body, peaceful mind and joyful Spirit. It is the same suggestions I give for Chair Yoga adaptions.

For Chair Yoga specifically, even if you have little or no physical movement ability, there are numerous benefits. This includes the calming of the nervous system and mind (from yogic breathing exercises and mantras), the social benefits (if practiced with others), as well as giving one a purpose, challenge and sense of accomplishment after practicing and doing something productive. Yoga is a discipline with great rewards.

What are the benefits of Chair Yoga?

Practicing yoga in chairs gives the same benefits as any other yoga practice does, relative to the practitioner's abilities and capabilities. Just like all yoga (when applied holistically and safely), Chair Yoga can give you more flexibility (in body and mind), physical and mental strength, improves balance, increases energy and vitality, improves memory and clarity and improves concentration. It can also improve overall feelings of wellness, including physical health, vitality and mental peace. Just taking time for yourself a few minutes a day to benefit your well-being can be an accomplishment in itself.

Who can practice Chair Yoga?

Everyone can do yoga! Chair Yoga is a safe and effective way to practice yoga at any age, stage and level of health, ability or mobility.

This includes practicing yoga:

- At work (at your desk)

- On airplanes

- With limited mobility

- For a gentle yoga practice

- With an acute or chronic illness

- Pre- and post surgery

- While healing from an injury

- In a wheelchair

- While pregnant

- In a hospital or rehab center

- In an assisted living home

- With a support group

- While healing from post-traumatic stress

Options are available for certain yoga postures to sit or stand (using the chair back as support if needed). If you are unable to do the standing version, you can do the upper body movements while seated, or modify it as you need to so that you are comfortable, safe and at ease. For those with limited physical mobility or energy limitations, the breathing exercises, mental concentration, and relaxation alone are enough without the physical exercises, so that truly: yoga is for everyone!

What do you wear for Chair Yoga?

Anything you want! This can make Chair Yoga more accessible to some than a yoga class at a studio or health club that may require a change of clothes and more time to prepare.

At work, you can do Chair Yoga in business attire and with shoes on. In general, however, it is advised to wear comfortable clothes you can stretch in, but it is not necessary. Yoga can be done in shoes, socks or bare feet. If the standing postures are practiced, please note that bare feet are preferable to avoid slipping. Keep in mind that yoga is not just about the physical exercises and postures alone, but it includes breathing and meditation. That can be done anywhere and anytime, starting with a slow, deep breath.

When do you practice Chair Yoga?

You can do Chair Yoga anytime and anywhere. Since the yoga practice includes breathing exercises, meditation and concentration exercises, you can even practice it in environments where you do not want to do active yoga postures and exercises. In fact, no one will even know you are practicing yoga except for the fact that they will see how much more calm, refreshed and content you may seem afterwards. Even one minute a day helps, so try it whenever and wherever you can.

If you want to establish a daily practice, which is recommended for progress, easing pain and discomfort, general wellness maintenance and even prevention of possible future aches and pains, consistent daily practice will produce the best results. However, do not be discouraged if your schedule, energy level or health prevents you from practicing Chair Yoga as much as you would like or intend to. Just start where you are with one minute a day and progress from there as you are able.

If you create the same time of day to practice, that will allow the mind and body to create a habit, so that less motivation and effort is required as time goes on to practice. That is because you will want to practice out of the experience of feeling better day to day when you do. However, be gentle with yourself if you miss a day and start again when you are able.

What type of chair do you use?

It is best to use a chair that is not on wheels, if it is available, for more stability. However at work or in an office or hospital setting, for example, use what is available but just be mindful to not slip if the chair is on wheels, or put the chair against a wall for more stability. This book uses the word "chair" which can be interchanged with how do yoga in a wheelchair, on a couch, on an airplane seat or in other settings when adapting traditional yoga postures is appropriate.

The chair in the yoga posture demonstrations in this book have an open back and are commonly found at yoga studios. However, some chairs have arms on the sides, which can be useful for spinal twists (to rest the arms). Try to get creative and adapt the ideas for doing yoga in a chair as best you can based on the space and chairs that you have available.

The remaining chapters of this book will include photos and descriptions of Chair Yoga adaptions of yoga postures from my SunLight Chair Yoga: yoga for everyone! book. You can try the Chair Yoga ideas for poses that are not comfortable otherwise. Chair Yoga is also useful to try at your desk, as a quick break from the computer, or while traveling (on an airplane). Yoga is for everyone!

Time to practice!

"Practice and all is coming." Pattabhi Jois, Ashtanga Yoga

"The ultimate goal of yoga is to always observe things accurately, and therefore never act in a way that will make us regret our actions later." TKV Desikachar

Yoga Practice

3

In Chapter 3, Yoga Practice

- Yoga practice contents
- Tips for new students
- Centering
- Mantras
- Warm-ups
- San Salutations
- Yoga postures
- Restorative Yoga

The components of a well-rounded yoga practice include:

- Centering (base posture, breathing and tuning in with *mantras*)
- Warm-ups (joint warm-ups and/or Sun Salutations, *Surya Namaskar*)
- Yoga exercises
- Postures (*asanas*)
- Yogic breathing practices *(pranayama)*
- Relaxation *(savasana)*
- Meditation (*dhyana*)
- Closing chants *(mantras)*

This chapter shows options for a Hatha Yoga practice (with and without a chair), Gentle Yoga and Chair Yoga options for each pose or practice. Find which one is best for your needs, so that the practice is comfortable and easeful, so that the body and mind can relax deeply. Even if the body is working strongly in a posture, focus on the breath and relaxing the muscles. You do not need to hold the posture longer than is comfortable. Yoga is a way to integrate the body and mind. The *yoga sutras* is a text that states the yoga asana should be comfortable and steady, or relaxed but firm (in Sanskrit *sthira sukham asanam).*

Keep in mind that the Yoga Sutras have 196 verses, of which that verse mentioned above, and only one other, talk about the yoga postures. Verse 2.47 says in Sanskrit *prayatna shaithilya ananta samapattibhyam,* which means that the way master the yoga posture is to relax or lessen tension and to meditate/merge with the Infinite. Verse 2.48 says in Sanskrit *tatah dvandva anabhighata,* which means once the postures are mastered, there will be freedom from disturbances from the pairs of opposites (such as hot and cold, good and bad, pleasure and pain).

Yoga is about finding the stillness in the mind. As you practice the yoga exercises for physical health, vitality, flexibility, mobility, balance and strength, keep this in mind if you ever get discouraged with the physical practice. Yoga is so much more than the yoga *asana* and postures, although yoga *asana* by itself is still so helpful.

So let's begin. As the Yoga Sutra 1.1 says *Atha Yoganushasanam,* which translates to: "now let the study of yoga begin" or "now begins the scientific discipline of yoga".

Yoga Practice Contents:

To start a home practice, after a few warm ups and Sun Salutations, try one pose or practice from each type of posture (a forward bend, an inversion, a backbend, a spinal twist, etc.) For a full practice, try the chapter on the Sivananda Yoga sequence, either as a Chair Yoga adapted practice of the full Hatha Yoga practice, which includes the Sun Salutations as a warm up and 12 main yoga *asanas,* followed by deep relaxation. Modify the practice to meet your needs, for duration and intensity.

A sample 10-minute yoga sequence

- 1 minute Centering
- 3 minutes Warm-ups (Sun Salutes or Joint Warm-ups)
- 4 minutes Yoga *Asanas*
- 2 minutes Relaxation
- Chanting (3 *Aum's* or *Shanti*)

A sample 30-minute yoga sequence

- 3 minutes Centering
- 5 minutes Warm-ups (Sun Salutations or Joint Warm-ups)
- 15 minutes Yoga *Asanas*
- 7 minutes Relaxation
- Closing Mantras

Sivananda Yoga 90 minute sequence

- Pranayama (Breathing Exercises)
- Sun Salutations (Warm Ups 3-6 Rounds)
- Headstand *(Sirshasana) or* Child's Pose
    - *(Balasana)* and/or Dolphin Pose
- Shoulderstand *(Sarvangasana)*
    - Or Legs up on the Wall or Chair Pose
- Plough *(Halasana)*
- Fish *(Matsyasana)*
- Forward bend *(Paschimothanasana)*
- Cobra *(Bhujangasana)*
- Locust *(Shalabhasana)*
- Bow *(Dhanurasana)*
- Spinal Twist (*Ardha Matsyendrasana)*
- Crow pose *(Kakasana)* or Tree Pose (*Vrksasana)*
- Standing Forward Bend *(Pada Hasthasana)*
- Triangle *(Trikonasana)*
- *Corpse Pose (Savasana)*
    - *Autosuggestion and Deep Relaxation*

Elements of a Yoga Practice

Warm Ups

Sun Salutations

Side Bends

Inversions

Forward Bends

Backbends

Spinal Twists

Balance Poses

Relaxation

Breathing Exercises

Meditation

Mantras

Tips for new students

Yoga is not the same as exercise as you may know it. The yoga exercises are to be done in a way that is a gentle, comfortable and relaxing practice for your body and mind. Even if the muscles of the body are working hard, it is more beneficial and recommended to only go as far as you are comfortable and to take breaks as needed. Especially if you are healing from an injury or dealing with certain aches and pains, make sure the yoga is easing them, or at least not aggravating any preexisting condition or injury.

Yoga postures, called "asanas" in Sanskrit, are defined by the Yoga Sutras of Patanjali, as a steady but comfortable seat for meditation. It also says "posture is mastered by releasing tension and meditating on the Infinite or Unlimited." (Yoga Sutra 2.47) Based on that, for the maximum benefit, make sure that the body is comfortable in all yoga postures and exercises. Some of the movements in this book are modified from the classic yoga postures and others are created for the modern age.

Please consult your doctor or medical provider for any questions or concerns for specific illnesses, ailments or injuries or any other health concerns, especially if you are not sure what you can and cannot do. For prenatal modifications, only do what is comfortable. Consult your doctor about any additional questions. Most postures in this book are safe for all trimesters, except spinal twists, inversions and postures lying on the stomach or back. If you are pregnant, modify as directed by your physician. For example, you can twist from the upper body only (the shoulders, neck and head) vs. from the spine as usually practiced.

A yoga class or practice class can help you to develop balance, well-being and peace of mind. It can teach you simple stretches and yoga postures for health, breathing exercises for mental calm, and relaxation techniques to enhance your well-being. You can also learn how to increase flexibility, ease neck, shoulder and back tension and improve balance and concentration. You can find a teacher that offers modifications if you are pregnant, injured or have any health conditions that you aren't sure how to modify for from a book alone.

10 Simple Points to Keep in Mind as you Practice:

1. In yoga class or on your own, only do the postures or exercises that are comfortable.

2. There should be no pain in the joints or body during the practice.

3. Modify postures or rest as needed.

4. If you have a pre existing injury that is aggravated by a certain movement or exercises please notify the yoga instructor right away.

5. Check with your doctor for any concerns from prior conditions or injuries if you are not sure what you can and cannot do.

6. Yoga is not competitive. Go at your own pace.

7. We are all unique- do what is comfortable for your body in each practice.

8. "No pain, no pain." We do yoga to ease pain in the body, not to create more. Be gentle even if you want a challenge.

9. Ask the instructor for modifications if pregnant, injured, ill or needing a different way to do a pose than is suggested.

10. Enjoy the practice! This is not about right or wrong, winning or losing but to feel better in the body and gain more peace in the mind.

Getting Started

Centering

It's important to start the practice with a few moments, or minutes of stillness, awareness and observation. This way you can see the state of your body, mind, emotions and energy level before starting the practice, which is often useful to guide your practice as well as to compare your state of being after the practice. This enables you to feel yoga's benefits each time you practice.

Centering is also a way to create a sacred space, even if practicing a few minutes at work. This brief 'pause' before starting the yoga exercises also gives your mind a transition from the worldly activities and external focuses, to bring attention to your inner world. It is the inner world in yoga practice that you want to start to observe so that we can find the peace within.

It is helpful to establish a comfortable physical yoga posture (yoga *asana*) before practicing the breathing, concentration or chants to focus and calm the mind. Start sitting tall. Following are some options for a comfortable seat, including sitting in a cross-legged seat on the ground or in a chair.

Easy Pose, *Sukhasana*

Sit tall on the floor with the legs crossed. Allow the head to be centered over the spine. Sit on a folded towel or blanket if you need support. If the knees are higher than the hips or if it is difficult to sit tall, sit on a cushion, folded towel or blanket. Relax the legs, the face and the shoulders. Take a few slow, deep breaths and allow your mind to get centered. Bring awareness to the present moment. Feel the body. Observe the breath.

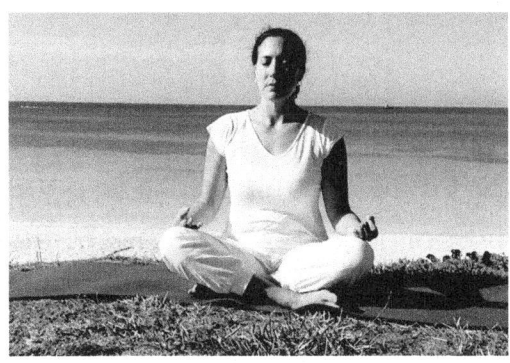

Affirmations: I am centered. I am present.

Chair Yoga Easy Pose, *Sukhasana*

Sit tall in your chair with the feet hip-width apart and the heels under the knees. Point the toes forward. Sit tall, away from the chair back, from the base of the spine through the top of the head. Rest the hands on the thighs. Take a few slow, deep breaths to get centered. Bring your awareness to the present moment. Inhale as you lift the spine and exhale as you relax in the posture. Relax your shoulders, your jaw and your eyes. Go through your body to check for areas that are holding on to physical tension (called a "body scan"). Let go of tension as you exhale.

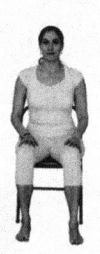

Benefits: Gives the mind time to pause and get centered. Feeling the feet on the ground (earth) helps balance the mental energies to feel less scattered and more 'grounded' or rooted.

<u>Affirmation</u>: I am centered

Easy Pose With Prayer Hands,
Sukhasana with Hands in Anjali Mudra

Sitting tall in Easy Pose, place your hands together in a prayer pose in the center of your chest, called *Anjali Mudra*. This is a devotional hand posture. Place your thumbs on your sternum (chest bone). Relax your shoulders. Allow the head to bow slightly towards the heart area or just close the eyes close as you bring awareness to the heart area. Tune into your inner teacher and inner guide. This can be your breath, your intuition, or inner wisdom.

Photo: Anjali Mudra in Easy Pose

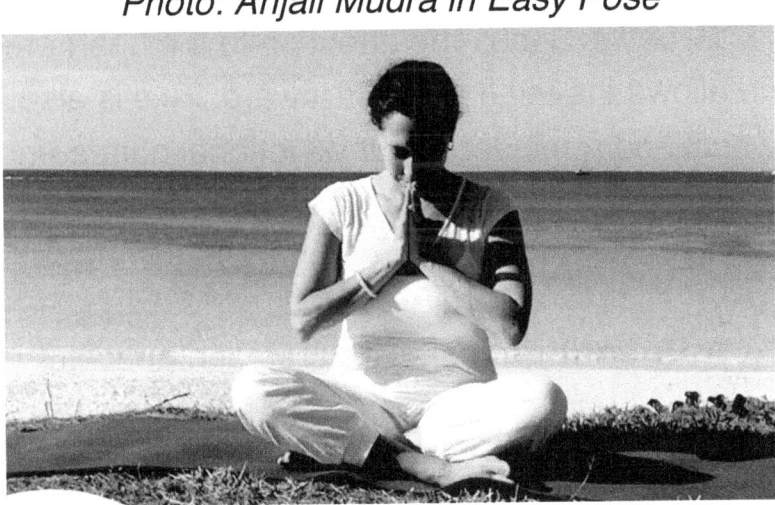

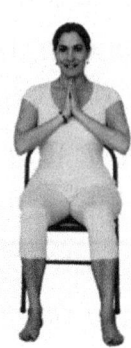

Anjali Mudra in Chair Yoga Easy Pose

Benefits: Brings the attention to the heart area and allows the mind to focus inward. This is also a symbol and reminder of our devotional nature and perhaps reminds us to take a moment to feel grateful and connected to our inner truth.

Affirmations: I am centered and peaceful.

Tuning in With Mantras

If you resonate to do so, you can also tune in with a simple Sanskrit mantra. A mantra is a repetitive sound, or mind projection of a sound current that the mind can associate with a positive, calming or uplifting image or vibration. The yogic sound currents allow the mind to shift from the busyness and business of the day to the inner world where peace and tranquility reside. A simple mantra to tune in with can be the Universal Mantra "AUM". Inhale deeply. As you exhale, chant AUM (OM) 3x silently or out loud. Allow the sound to wash away all of your worries and thoughts of the world. Chant *shanti* as listed below which means peace in Sanskrit. Tune in to the inner peace deep inside.

AUM (OM) 3X, Aum Shanti Shanti Shanti,

Translation: *Aum Peace Peace Peace*

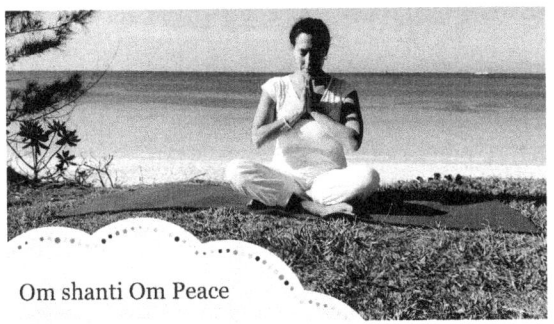

Om shanti Om Peace

Although the *mantras* from India are in Sanskrit

or Gurmukhi languages, and are said to be divine sounds that were spoken from the past seers and saints of India, with many benefits connecting us to ancient lineages of yoga, there is also a benefit to chanting an uplifting or peaceful word in your own language or language of choice. Be mindful to use words and sounds that create a calming effect on the mind. After the chant, take a moment or more to sit in stillness and observe the effects of the mantra or sound current. Some other ideas to chant are below:

Shalom Shalom Shalom

Translation: *Peace Peace Peace*

If you prefer you can also create your own affirmation that brings the mind to inner peace, such as:

Peace is in me. Peace is within.

For more in depth Sanskrit chants and invocations, try the chants on the following pages.

Om Namah Shivaye Gurave

Om Namah Shivaya Gurave

Saccidananda Murtaye

Nisprapancaya Shantaya

Niralambaya Tejase

Translation: I offer myself to the True Teacher within and without (the teacher of all teachers), who is united in Truth, Consciousness and Bliss, who is never absent and is peaceful, independent in its existence, and radiant.

Gayatri Mantra -Om Bhur Bhuvah Svah

Om Bhur Bhuvah Swaha

Tat Savitur Varenyam

Bhargo Devasya Dhi Mahi

Dhiyo Yo Nah Prachodayat

Translation: Om I meditate on the radiant and most venerable light of the divine, which issues forth the triple world, earth, ether, and cosmos. May the divine light illuminate and guide my intelligence.

Shantipat

Om saha navavatu

Saha nau bhunaktu

Saha viryam karavavahai

Tejasvi navadhitam astu

Ma vidvishavahi

Om shanti, shanti, shanti

Translation:

May we be protected together.

May we be nourished together.

May we work together with great vigor.

May our study be enlightening.

May there be no hatred between us.

Om peace, peace, peace.

Shanti Mantra (Peace Mantra)

sarvesham svastir bhavatu

sarvesham shantir bhavatu

sarvesham purnam bhavatu

sarvesham mangalam bhavatu

May there be well-being for all,

May there be peace for all.

May there be wholeness for all,

May there be happiness for all.

Yoga Postures *(Asanas)*
Standing Mountain Pose, *Tadasana*

Stand with the feet together or hip width apart for more stability. Balance the weight equally on both feet and allow the arms to rest along side the body. Feel the feet rooting into the earth, like a mountain base, as the top of the head rises towards the sky, like the mountaintop. Take a few slow, deep breaths.

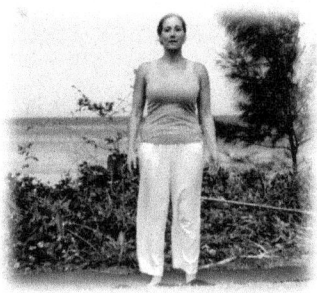

Benefits: Increases concentration, balance and stability, and gives the mind time to pause and get centered. Feeling the feet on the ground (earth) helps balance the mental energies to feel less scattered and feel more 'grounded' or rooted. This posture can be the first pose done before other standing postures.

Affirmations: I am balanced. I am grounded. I feel connected to the earth and to my body.

Chair Yoga Standing Mountain Pose,
Tadasana

Stand behind the chair with the feet hip-width apart with the hands on the chair top, alongside the body, or in *Anjali Mudra* (palms in Prayer Pose). Have the toes pointing forward. Align the head so that it is centered over the spine. Balance the weight equally between the right and left foot. Hold and breathe for a few rounds.

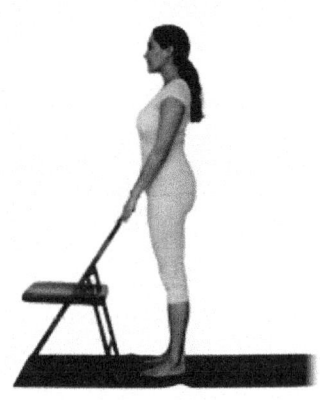

Affirmations: I am balanced. I am centered.

Chair Yoga Seated Mountain Pose,
Tadasana

Sit tall in your chair with the feet hip-width apart and your heels under the knees. The toes point forward. If comfortable, sit away from the chair back and lift from the base of your spine through top of the head. Allow the hands to rest on the thighs. This is the same posture as Easy Pose, when practicing in a chair.

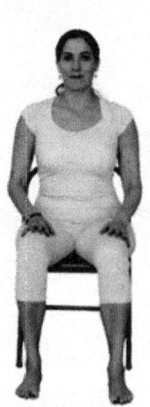

Benefits: Improves posture and focus.

Affirmation: I am centered.

As variation in Mountain Pose, place the palms in Prayer Pose for Equal Standing Pose, as in the photos below.

Equal Standing Pose, *Samasthiti*

(Mountain Pose with Anjali Mudra)

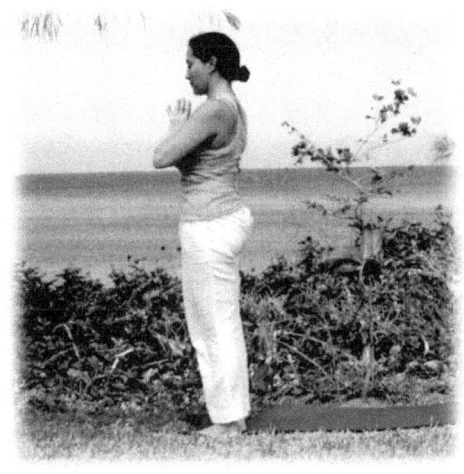

Chair Yoga Seated, *Samasthitihi*

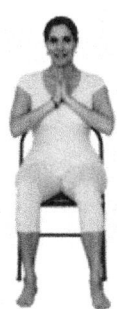

Chair Yoga Equal Standing Pose,
Samasthiti

From Mountain Pose, place the hands together in Prayer Pose, if you feel stable and balanced without the chair. Hold and breathe slow and deep for 5 rounds.

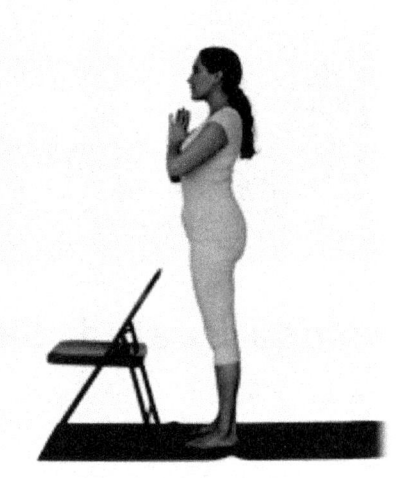

Benefits: Improves balance and centers the mind.

Affirmations: I am balanced. I am centered.

Yoga for Everyone!

Warming Up the Body

The warms-ups are done to increase circulation, and mobility in the joints of the body, before practicing other yoga postures *(asanas)*. The warm-ups by itself however, can also be a beneficial practice and perhaps all that is needed for certain conditions or energy levels. For example, if you are waiting for a surgery, healing an injury or illness, or managing a chronic illness, 5-10 minutes of joint warm-ups may be enough for the body on some days as the only exercise. It can be followed by relaxation and breathing practices or meditation, which is more restful. For some, the joint warm-ups may not be needed, if the body feels comfortable to start with a gentle or full yoga Sun Salutation. There is no right or wrong order to practice these warm ups. Try one of them, a few or all of them. There is no set order to practice them in either. Be creative.

Warm-ups can be done standing, lying down for a Gentle Yoga practice, or seated as in the Chair Yoga photos below. They can also be useful to warm the body up before a vigorous Hatha Yoga practice (standing postures, lying down and seated postures, inversions and balancing poses).

Wrist Rotations

Rotate your hands around your wrists 3 to 6x. Make circles in the air with your fingers. Make circles with closed fists or open hands. Reverse directions and repeat 3 to 6x.

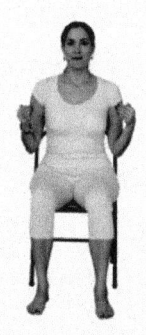 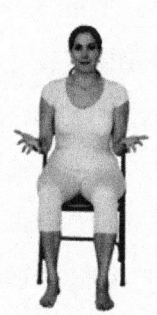

Photo (left): Fingers Inwards

Photo (right): Circling Away

Benefits: Improves the range of motion in the wrist joints. Increases the ability to adapt to changes when getting up from chairs, out of bed, etc. Eases wrist strain from computer use.

Point and Flex Foot Movements

Lift both feet a few inches off the ground. Slowly point your toes towards the floor then gently pull your toes back towards you 5 to 8x.

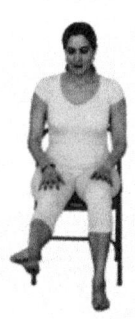 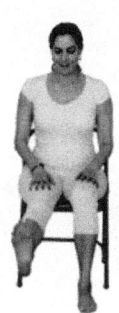

Photo left: Foot Flexed   Photo right: Toes Pointed

Benefits: Improves the range of motion in the ankles. This can be done at your desk, on airplanes, on the couch or in a wheelchair.

Ankle Rotations

Ankle Rotations Lying Down

Lie on your back with the knees bent and the feet hip width apart, as in the photo below. Let the feet rest on the ground. Hug one knee into the chest. Rotate the ankle a few times in each direction. Switch sides.

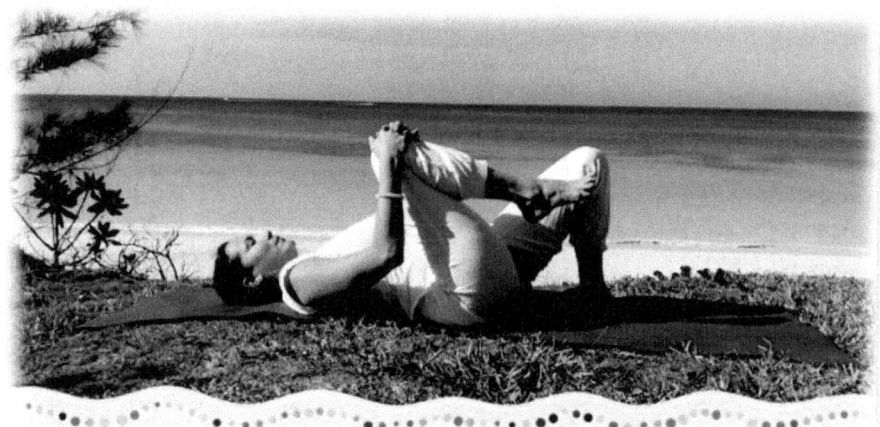

Knee to Chest with Ankle Rotations

Benefits: Improves the range of motion in the ankles. The lying down version is useful for those feeling fatigued and needing a more restful posture to practice the joint warm-ups.

Yoga for Everyone!

Standing Ankle Rotations

Stand behind a chair with the toes pointing forward and the feet hip width apart. Place the hands on the top of the chair back for support. Lift one heel (or foot) and rotate one foot around the ankle 3 to 6x. Make circles in the air with your big toe. Reverse directions and then switch sides.

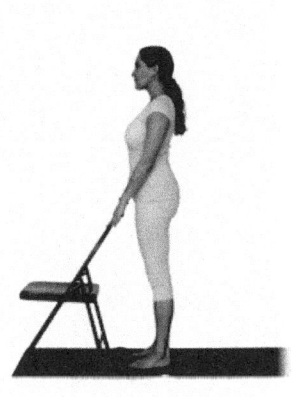

Benefits: Improves the range of motion and balance in the feet and ankles and the ability to adapt to changes when getting up from chairs, out of bed, etc. This can help to increase the circulation in the legs and feet. It helps to ease the joints on flights or during long meetings or days at your desk. The standing version strengthens the legs and increases balance.

Chair Yoga Seated Ankle Rotations

Rotate your feet around your ankles 3 to 6x. Make circles in the air with your big toes. Make circles with one foot at a time or with both feet together at the same time. Reverse directions and repeat 3 to 6x. Then rotate one foot clockwise and the other counterclockwise. Switch sides.

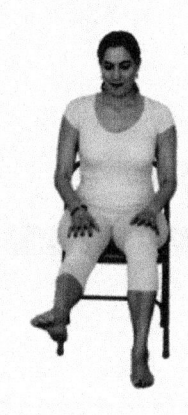

Benefits: Improves the range of motion in the ankles. This can be done at your desk, on airplanes, on the couch or in a wheelchair.

Prayer Pose Wrists Warm Ups in
Anjali Mudra

Sitting cross-legged on the floor or in a chair (as in the photo on the following page), place your hands together in prayer position in front of the heart area. Place your thumbs on your sternum. Relax your shoulders. Sit tall and focus at the heart area.

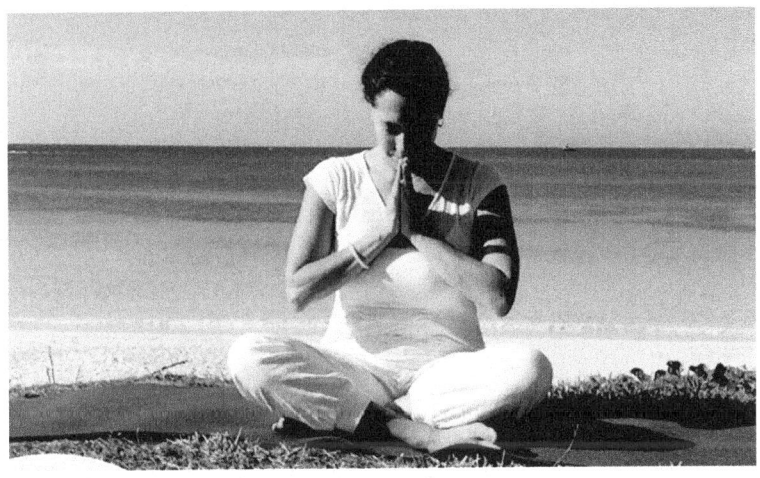

Benefits: This brings the attention to the heart area and allows the mind to focus inward. This is also a symbol and reminder of our devotional nature and reminds us to take a moment to feel grateful and perhaps faithful.

Prayer Pose Exercises

1- Rotations: Bring your palms into Prayer Pose. Rotate your fingers towards your heart, then towards the floor in front of you. Repeat 5x.

2- Push Hands: In Prayer Pose, push your hands from side to side. Feel resistance from the hand you are pushing into.

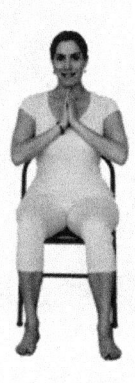

Photo: Prayer Pose (Anjali Mudra)

Benefits: Warms up and loosens the wrists. This eases strain from computer use or repetitive movements and for those sitting long hours at a desk.

Affirmations: I am grateful. I feel purposeful.

Sacred Circles

Sacred Circles can be done from a cross-legged seat (Easy Pose) or sitting in a chair, as in the photos shown on the following page. From Prayer Pose, inhale and stretch the hands up, keeping your palms together. Exhale as you separate the hands away from each other and draw a big circle around you. Inhale as you join the palms back to Prayer Pose at the navel center and stretch the arms up again. Repeat 5 to 8x. See the photos on the following page.

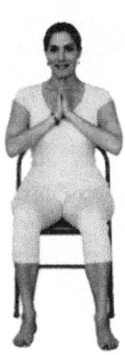

Sacred Circles

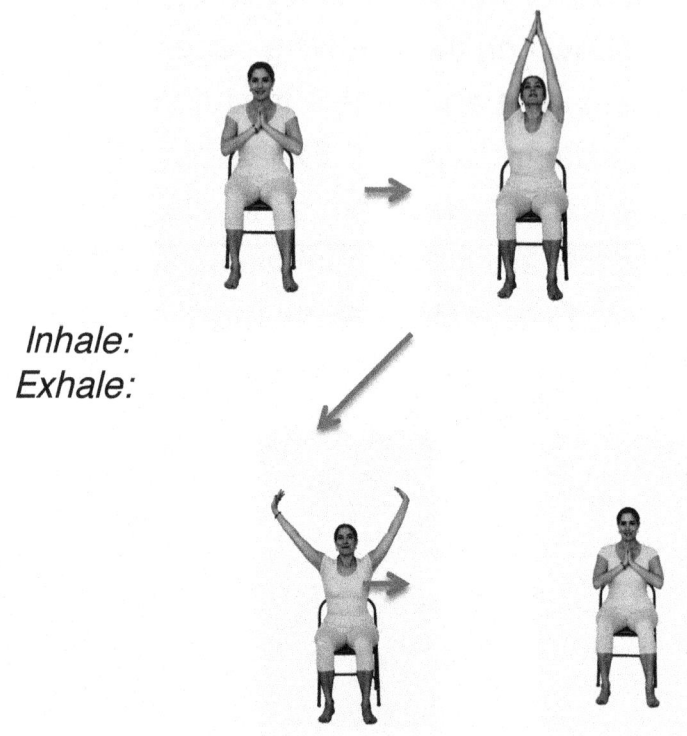

Inhale:
Exhale:

    Benefits: Warms up and loosens the upper back and shoulders, increases circulation and stretches the hands and arms (good for computer use and for those sitting long hours at a desk). Imagine you're pushing away any negativity or energies you don't need. Also, this coordinates the breath with the body for mental calming and soothing of the nervous system. This can be done before any yoga practice or by itself as a one-minute stretch break while at work.

Reverse Namaste

Bring your hands behind the back. Hold on to your elbows or wrists or fingers. If you are able, place the palms in prayer position behind your back. Take 3 to 5 slow, deep breaths as you feel the upper back and shoulders opening.

Reverse Sacred Circles

Inhale and stretch the hands up with the palms facing skyward. Exhale as you bring the palms to Prayer Pose overhead and then to the sternum (chest bone). Repeat 5-8x. See the photos on the following page.

Benefits: Warms up and loosens the upper back and shoulders, increases circulation and stretches the hands and arms (good for computer use and for those sitting long hours at a desk), and coordinates the breath with the body for mental calming. You can imagine you are gathering energy *(prana)* with your hands.

Affirmations: I am protected. I release that which no longer serves me. I invite in new, fresh *prana*, energy and positivity with every breath.

Reverse Sacred Circles

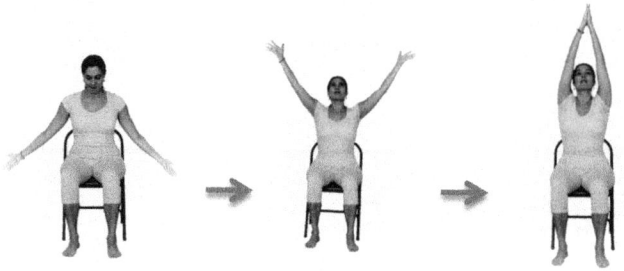

Inhale Arms Up Overhead   *Exhale Arms*

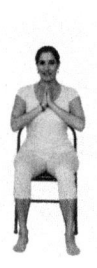
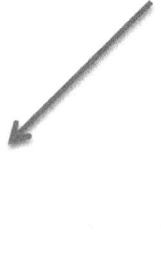

Prayer Pose

Benefits: Warms up and loosens the upper back and shoulders, increases circulation and stretches the hands and arms (good for computer use and for those sitting long hours at a desk), and coordinates the breath with the body for mental calming. You can imagine you are gathering energy *(prana)* with your hands.

Cat Cow Poses

Start in Table Pose, on all fours. Place the hands under the shoulders and the knees under the hips.

Cow Pose, *Bitilasana*:

Inhale as you lift the head and tailbone, allowing the heart to melt between the shoulder blades and relaxing the navel center towards the earth.

Cat Pose, *Marjaiasana:*

Exhale as you round the back, relaxing the neck. Keep the fingers stretched out on the floor evenly. This posture releases back and shoulder tensions and is a great way to release your neck and back after a long day at your desk.

Cat Cow Pose

Inhale as move into Cat Pose. Exhale as you shift to Cow Pose. Repeat 4 to 8x. See the photos on the following page.

Cat Cow

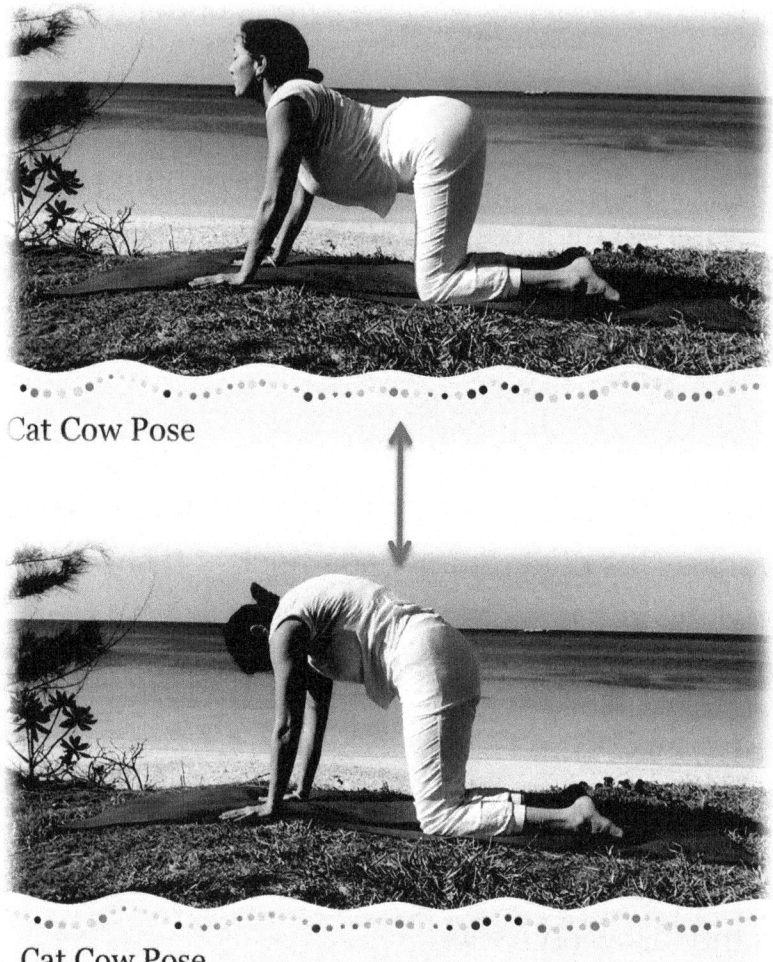

Cat Cow Pose

Cat Cow Pose

Benefits: Stretches the abdomen and back.
Relieves back tension.

Chair Yoga Cat Cow, *Marjaiasana to Bitilasana*

From Mountain Pose, inhale as you lift the heart into an upper back bend, sliding the hands towards the hips. Exhale as you round at the navel point (belly button) and round the upper back, reaching the hands towards the knees. You can also keep the arms straight with the hands above the knees for both poses. Keep the head centered. Repeat 4 to 8x. Feel the spine move like a wave in a meditative, rhythmic motion.

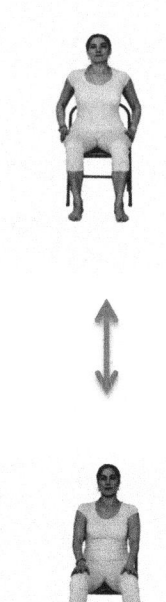

Inhale Cow
Exhale Cat

Benefits: Warms up the spine, eases back tension and increases energy.

Spinal Circles, "Sufi Grind" (modified from Kundalini Yoga)

Sit tall, either cross-legged on the ground, or sitting tall on your chair. If you are in a chair, have the feet hip width apart. Inhale as you lean slightly back and to the right. Then exhale as you lean forward and to the left. Continue moving the spine in a circular direction, keeping the head upright. Repeat 5x: inhale as you lean back and exhale as you lean forward. Reverse direction. See photos below.

Benefits: Warms up the spine, hips and back, eases back tension, coordinates the breath with the body and mind and increases energy.

Spinal Circles in Easy Pose

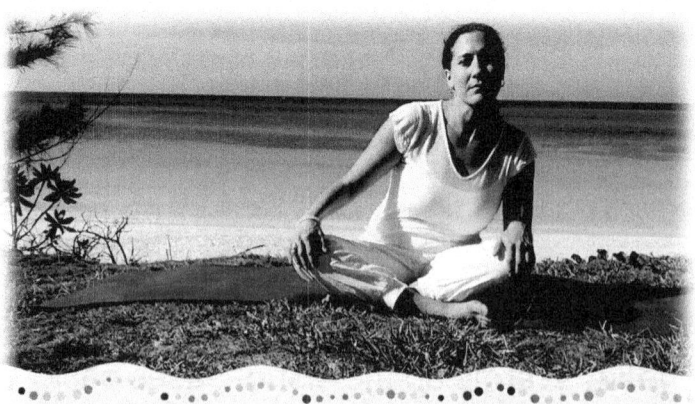

Spinal Circles

Yoga for Everyone!

Chair Yoga Spinal Circles

Sit tall in your chair with the feet hip-width apart. Inhale as you lean slightly back and to the right. Then exhale as you lean forward and to the left. Continue moving the spine in a circular direction, keeping the head upright. Repeat 5x: inhale as you lean back and exhale as you lean forward. Reverse direction.

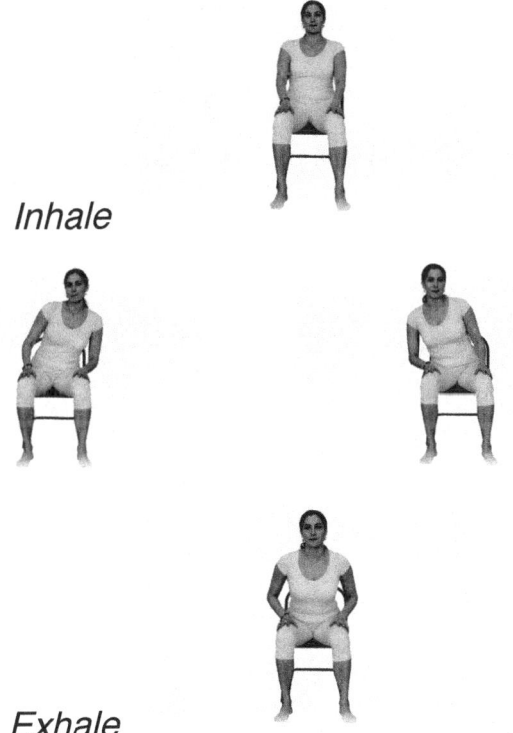

Inhale

Exhale

Benefits: Warms up the spine, hips and back, eases back tension, coordinates the breath with the body and mind and increases energy.

Shoulder Shrugs

Sitting cross-legged in Easy Pose or sitting tall in a chair, inhale as you shrug the shoulders up to the ears. Exhale as you drop the shoulders down, away from the ears. Imagine that you are releasing all your tensions and worries with each exhalation. Repeat 3 to 6x.

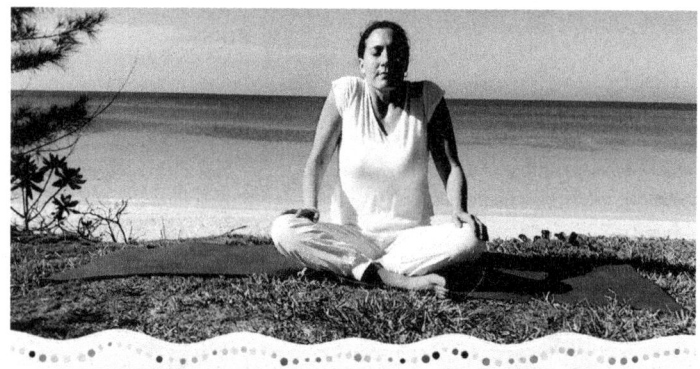

Shoulder Shrugs

Benefits: Eases neck and shoulder tensions and relaxes the trapezius muscle. This pose reminds the shoulders and upper back muscles to relax while on the computer or from general stress. This is also helpful to relax the neck and shoulders to relax on airplanes or on long road trips.

Affirmations: I am relaxed. I let go with ease.

Yoga for Everyone!

Shoulder Rolls and Movements

1- Circle the shoulders forward 5 to 10x. Reverse direction. Move with your breath. For example, inhale when the shoulders are up and exhale when they are down.

2- Bring the hands to shoulders and make circles with your elbows: small circles at first and then bigger circles. Reverse direction, 5 to 10x each. Move with your breath. For example, inhale when the elbows are up and exhale when the elbows are down.

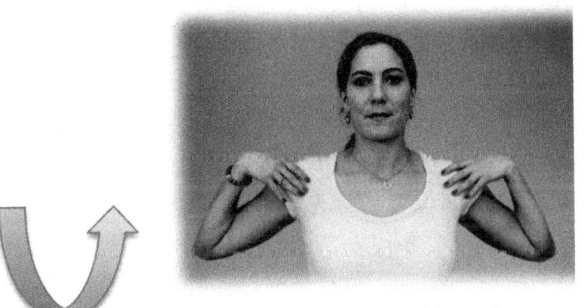

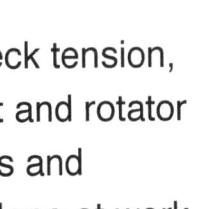

With Hands on Shoulders

Benefits: Eases shoulder and neck tension, increases mobility to the shoulder joint and rotator cuff, increases circulation and expands and relaxes the upper chest. This can be done at work or on an airplane for quick shoulder relief.

Neck Stretch

Inhale as you sit tall and center your head (from a cross-legged seat or sitting tall on a chair). Exhale as you lower your left ear to your left shoulder. The opposite hand can stretch towards the earth. Keep the shoulders relaxed. Switch sides. Repeat 5x in each direction or hold and breathe for 1-5 rounds of slow, deep breath.

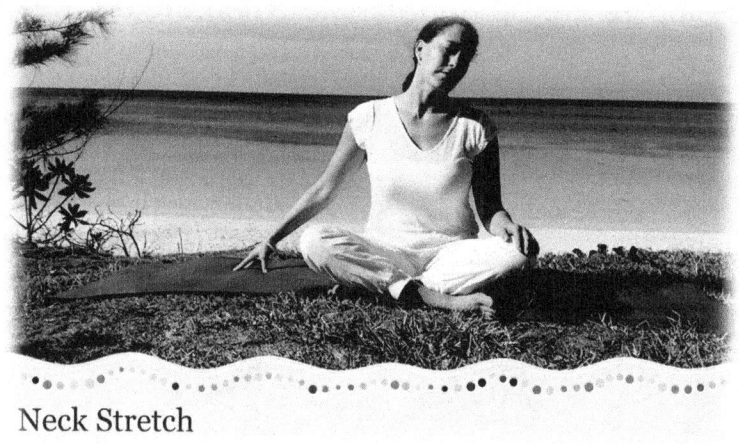

Neck Stretch

Benefits: Eases neck tension and stretches the sides of the neck.

Neck Rotations

Sitting tall in a chair, or cross-legged on the floor, turn your head side to side. Inhale as you bring your head to the center. Exhale as you turn your head to one side, looking over your shoulder as far as you are comfortable. Relax the shoulders and jaw as you sit tall. Move your eyes to each side with the neck movements. Switch sides. Repeat 5x in each direction.

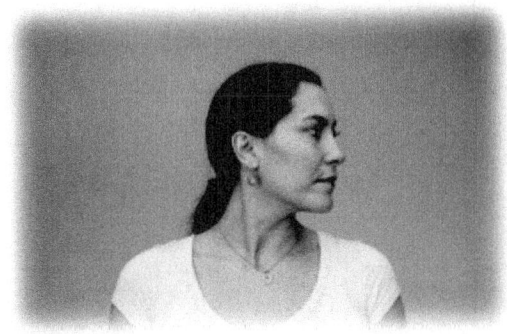

Benefits: Eases neck tension and brings mobility to the neck. Relieves computer-related neck tension or general dullness from lack of movement.

Half Neck Circles

Rotate the neck in half circles. Inhale as you lift one ear to your shoulder. Exhale as you bring the chin down towards your chest bone. Switch sides. Repeat 5x in each direction.

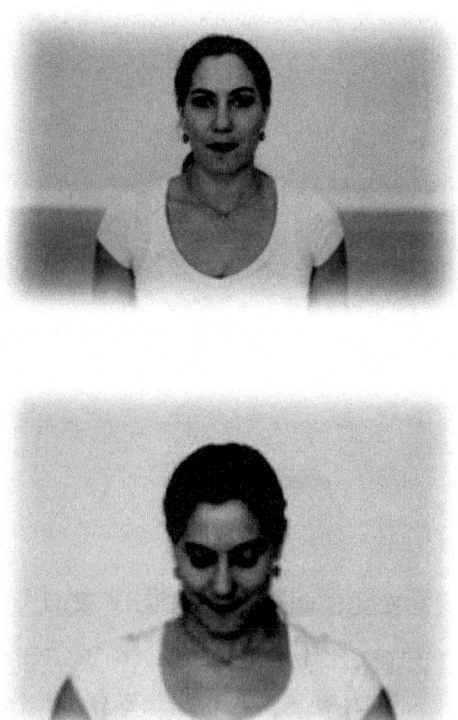

Benefits: Eases neck tension and brings mobility to the neck. This is useful on long flights or after computer use.

Full Neck Circles

Center the head over the spine. Draw 5 circles in the air with your nose. Inhale when the nose (chin) is up, and exhale when the nose (chin) comes down. Reverse directions.

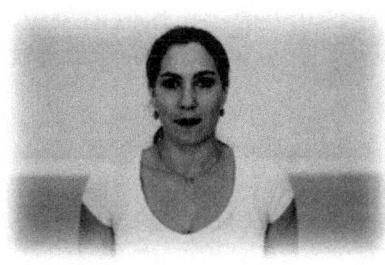

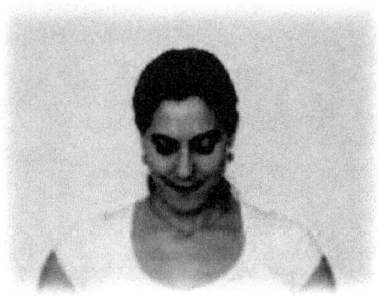

Photo: Full Neck Circles (position of the head is down as you exhale)

Benefits: Eases neck tension and increases neck joint mobility and range of motion. This is also useful on long flights or after computer use.

Precautions: For neck pain, move the eyes only.

Alternate Leg Raises, *Utanpadasana*

Lie on your back with the hands by the hips, or under the buttocks for more support. Inhale as you lift one leg up towards the sky, up to 90 degrees. Keep your opposite thigh on floor. Exhale as you lower. Switch legs. Repeat 5x on each side.

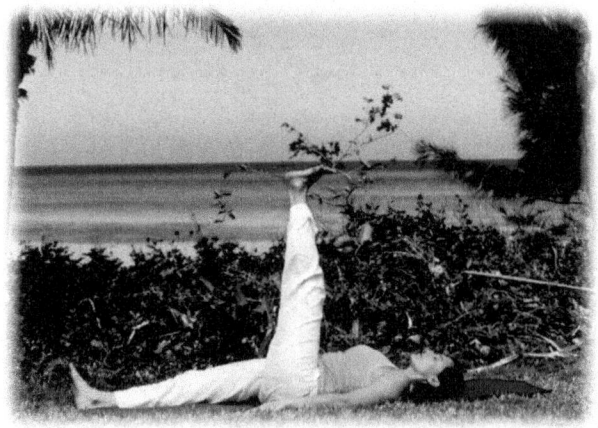

Benefits: Increases mobility in the hips, stretches the legs and strengthens the core and lower back.

Alternate Arm and Leg Raises

Lying on your back, bring both knees to the chest and the hands to the floor by the hips. Inhale as you lift one leg towards the sky and the opposite arm overhead. Exhale as you lower back to the starting position (both knees bent towards the chest with the hands on the floor by the hips). Switch sides, alternating 4-8 rounds.

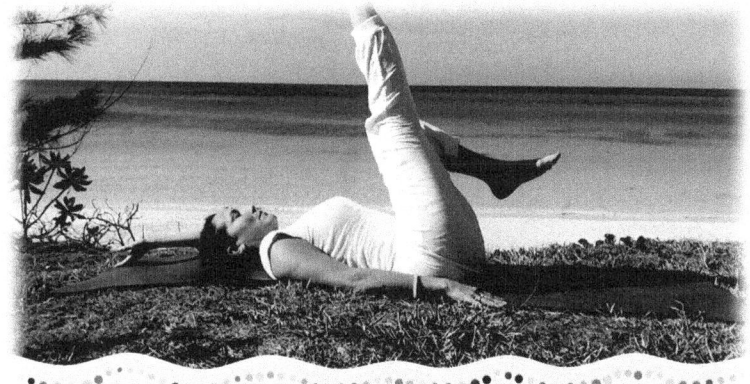

Alternate Arm and Leg Raises: opposite arm and leg

Benefits: Increases knee, hip, and shoulder joint mobility, improves circulation and is useful for right-left brain coordination.

Chair Yoga Alternate Leg Raises

Inhale as you lift one leg up (keep your thigh on the chair for support). Exhale as you lower. Switch legs. Repeat 5x on each side or as you are comfortable. Keep the back relaxed yet sitting tall.

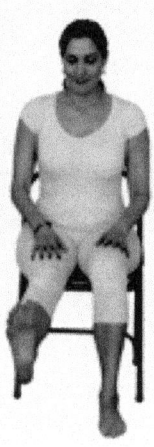

Benefits: Increases knee, hip, and shoulder joint mobility, improves circulation and is useful for right-left brain coordination.

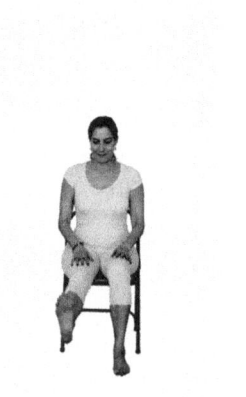

Inhale as you lift one foot/leg up (keep your thigh on the chair for support). Exhale as you lower. Switch legs. Repeat 5x on each side or as you are comfortable. Keep the back relaxed yet sitting tall.

Alternate Leg Raises

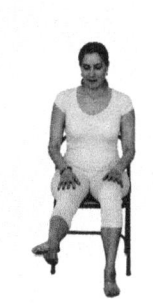

Point and Flex Variation: Inhale as you point the toes and raise the lower leg. Exhale as you and flex the foot and lower the leg. Repeat 3 to 5x. Switch sides. Reverse by flexing the foot as you inhale and lift, and pointing the toes as you exhale and lower. Repeat 5x. Switch sides.

Point and Flex

Benefits: Strengthens the quadriceps (muscles on the front of the thigh), helps the knee joint and stretches the legs. It brings circulation and energy to the legs and feet.

Upward Hand Pose, *Urdhva Hastasana*

Stretch the arms up overhead. Hold and breath for 1 to 5 slow, deep breathes.

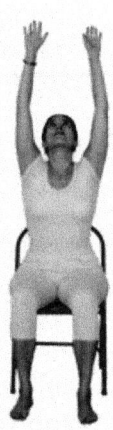

Benefits: Stretches the arms and waist and increases energy.

Single Arm Raises

Inhale as you lift one arm up overhead, as high as is comfortable for you. Exhale as you lower. Alternate arms. You can lower the arm to the side of the chair or to your lap. Repeat 5x on each side.

Double Arm Raises

Inhale as you lift both arms up overhead, as high as comfortable. Look up as you lift the arms to combine this with a neck movement. Exhale when you come down to lower the arms (and bring the head back to center if you were looking up). You can lower the arms to the side of the chair or to your lap. Repeat 5x.

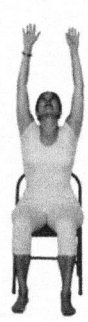

Benefits: Increases circulation and coordination. It also strengthens the arms, mind-body connection and breath awareness. Brings mobility to the shoulder joints and neck (if you add the head movements).

Precautions: For neck pain, keep the head centered and look up with the eyes only. For shoulder injuries bring the arms up to shoulder height or as far as comfortable.

Seated Chair Yoga Alternate Arm and Leg Raises

Inhale as you lift your right arm up, and extend the left leg out. Exhale as you lower the arm and leg. Switch sides and repeat 3 to 6x.

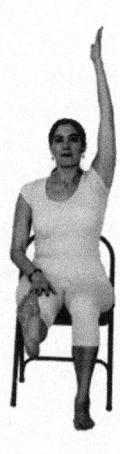

Benefits: Improves and increases coordination of the body and right and left sides of the brain, circulation, arm and leg mobility, range of motion in the shoulder and knee joints, and increases leg and arm strength. The seated Chair Yoga Leg Lifts also strengthens the quadriceps (muscles on the front of the thigh), helps the knee joint and stretches the legs.

Alternate Leg Raises, Point and Flex

Inhale as you point the toes and raise the lower leg. Exhale as you and flex the foot and lower the leg. Repeat 3 to 5x. Switch sides. Reverse by flexing the foot as you inhale and lift, and pointing the toes as you exhale and lower. Repeat 5x. Switch sides.

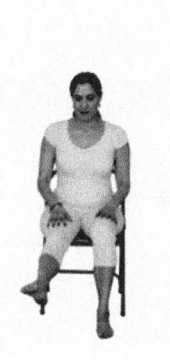 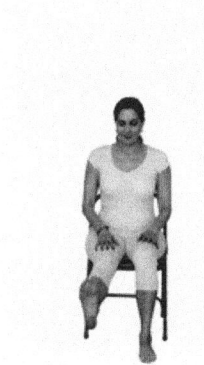

Benefits: Improves mobility and range of motion in the shoulder, knee and hip joint. The seated Chair Yoga Alternate Leg Lifts also strengthens the quadriceps (muscles on the front of the thigh), helps the knee joint and stretches the legs. It brings circulation and energy to the legs and feet.

Lying Down Knee Circles

Lying on your back, bring one knee to the chest. Hold behind the knee with the hands as in the photo below. Circle the knee in the air 3-6 rounds. Switch directions. Repeat with the other leg. You can also rotate the ankles while in this position after the knee circles,

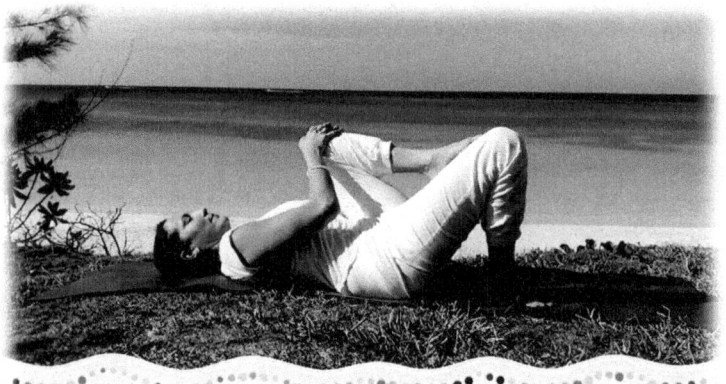

Knee to Chest to Knee Circles

Benefits: Increases knee mobility and can ease knee, hip, sciatic and low back pain.

Lying Down Circles (both knees)

Lying on your back, bring both knees to the chest. Hold behind the knees with the hands or place one hand on each knee, as in the photo below. Circle the both knees in the same direction for 3-6 rounds. Switch directions

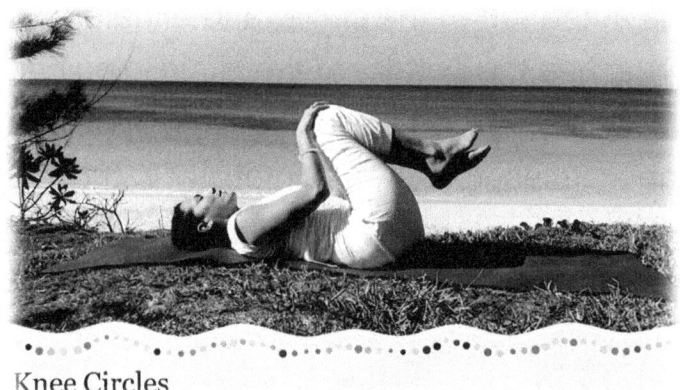

Knee Circles

Benefits: Increases mobility in the hip and knee joints, massages the back and eases pain or tension in the sciatic joint.

Chair Yoga Knee Circles

From Mountain Pose, lift one knee up and hold the leg behind the knee with hands as in the photo below. Make circles in the air with your knee. Repeat 5x. Reverse direction. Switch legs. Keep the spine tall. Relax the shoulders and jaw. The breathing is slow and deep. You can inhale as the knee is at the top of the circle, and exhale as the knee reaches the bottom of the circle. You can also rotate the ankles while in this position after the knee circles, to increase mobility in the joints.

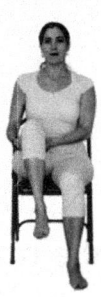

Benefits: Increases knee mobility and can ease knee, hip and low back pain. Strengthens the back muscles by keeping the spine tall.

Affirmations: I am flexible. I am relaxed.

Reflections

Take a few moments to pause and relax after practicing the warms ups. Pause and see how your body, mind and energy level feels afterwards. The warm ups alone can be repeated a few times as your main practice. Or continue your practice as you do some rounds of the Sun Salutations, as suggested on the following pages. Take a break and rest if you need. Go at your own pace. Yoga is for everyone!

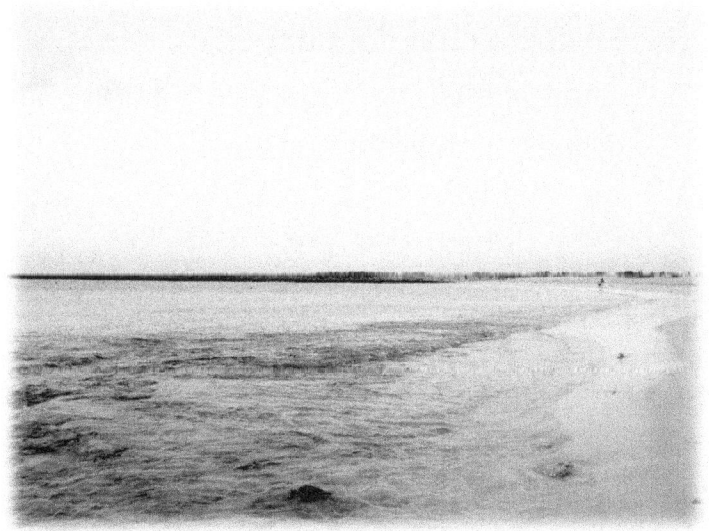

"Yoga teaches us to cure what need not be endured and endure what cannot be cured." B.K.S. Iyengar

Sun Salutations, *Surya Namaskar*

This section will offer four ways to practice the Sun Salutations:

- Sun Salutations (12 poses based on the Sivananda Yoga tradition)
- Gentle Yoga (gentle adaptations to the full Sun Salutation)
- Seated Chair Yoga Sun Salutations (using a chair for support)
- Standing Chair Yoga Sun Salutations (using a chair for support)

Sun Salutations *(Surya Namaskar)*

Sun Salutations are a series of yoga postures that flow together, moving with the rhythm of the breath. Traditionally, practiced at sunrise and sundown, facing the sun, they were done to honor the rising and setting of the sun and to generate heat in the body, improve flexibility and overall wellness. Sun Salutations also warms the body up for the main yoga postures, improves circulation, increases energy and vitality.

Without the sun we would not be here on earth. In India there is a mantra often chanted as the sun rises.

ॐ भूर्भुवः स्वः *Om Bhur bhuva swaha*

तत् सवितुर्वरेण्यं *Tat savitur Varenyam*

भर्गो देवस्य धीमहि *Bhargo Devasya Dhimahi*

hधियो यो नः प्रचोदयात् *Dhio yo nah Prachodayat*

"*AUM* -we realize ourselves as manifestation of the Three Worlds and the Beyond; we contemplate the Spiritual Sun that begins to manifest in us in its Perfect Form. We meditate on its Highest Light granting us Wisdom and Bliss. Let it enlighten us with the Light of its Truth." *Translation by the Sri Aurobindo Center of Integral Yoga

Some other mantras honoring the sun are mantras traditionally done with each move of the Sun Salutation. See the next two pages for each mantra and it's meaning.

Sun Salutation Mantras

Om Mitraaya Namaha Who is friendly to all

Om Ravaye Namaha The shining one, the radiant one

Om Suryaya Namaha Who dispels darkness and brings activity

Om Bhaanave Namaha One who is illuminated, bright one

Om Khagaya Namaha Who is all pervading, one who moves through the sky

Om Pooshne Namaha Giver of nourishment & fulfillment

Om Hiranyagarbhaaya Namah Who has a brilliant golden color

Om Mareechaye Namaha The giver of infinite rays of light

Producer of Everything

Om Aarkaaya Namaha One who is the Healer and inspires Awe in All

Om Bhaaskaraya Namaha Giver of wisdom and cosmic illumination

The sun sustains our planet. Without the sun, we would not exist on earth. Here, we can take time to honor the actual sun and to honor the elements of heat, warmth and energy within our bodies as well.

You can match the seated and standing Sun Salutations to the rhythm of the breath. If you need extra support standing, you can put a second chair in front of you, and one behind you for added assistance to your balance. You can do this as a flowing sequence with one breath per movement (as a moving meditation) or hold each posture for 3 to 5 deep breaths or as you feel comfortable. You can alternate between the seated and standing versions, as you need. When you are finished, sit quietly and relax for 5 to 8 slow, deep breaths. Observe the heart rate (which may speed up from Sun Salutations). Observe the temperature of the body (which may heat up from this sequence). Allow the heart and body to relax.

The benefits of the Sun Salutations are numerous, including increasing mobility, energy, flexibility, circulation and endurance at the beginning or middle of the day. It is also calming to unwind at the end of the day. It is most powerful when done at sunrise or sunset.

Sun Salutations, *Surya Namaskar*

Based on the Sivananda Yoga tradition

1. Stand tall with the feet together in Mountain Pose. Bring the hands together in Prayer Pose in front of the heart center. This posture is now called Equal Standing Pose. Press the feet down to the earth equally and press the hands together equally.

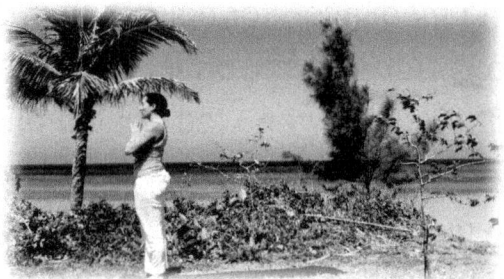

2. Inhale as you stretch the arms up overhead and slightly back, creating a backbend.

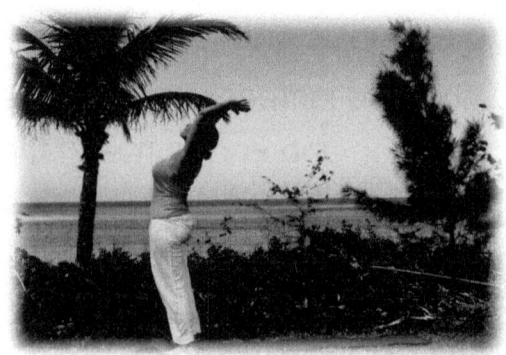

Yoga for Everyone!

3. Exhale as you bend forward. Touch the floor, with the hands along side the feet. Bend the knees if you need.

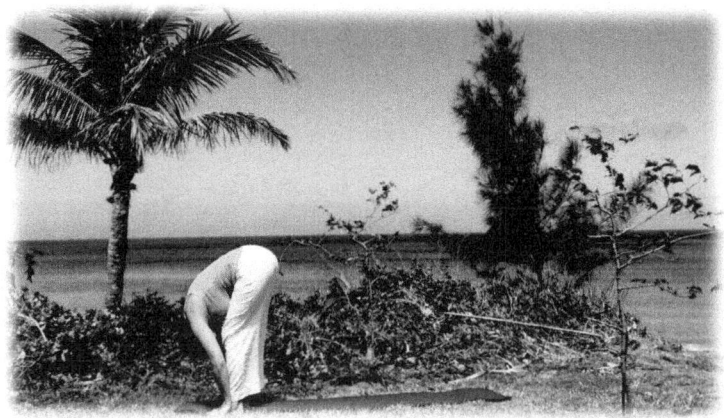

4. Inhale as you step the right leg back into Low Lunge Pose, lowering the knee to the floor.

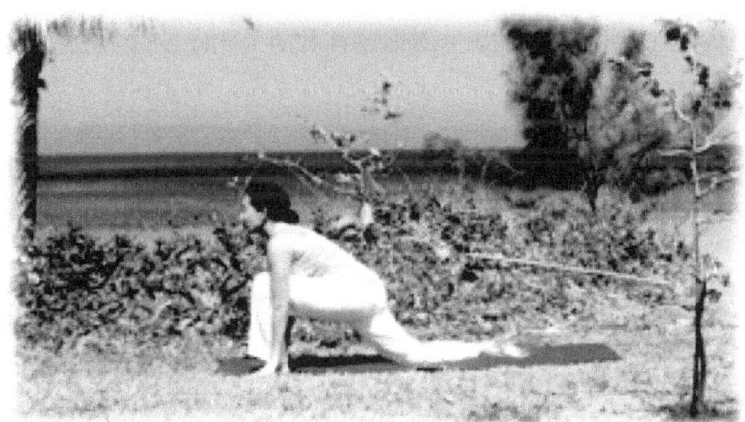

5. Step the left leg back into a Plank Pose, keeping the shoulders over the wrists and the legs strong and straight. Press the heels back.

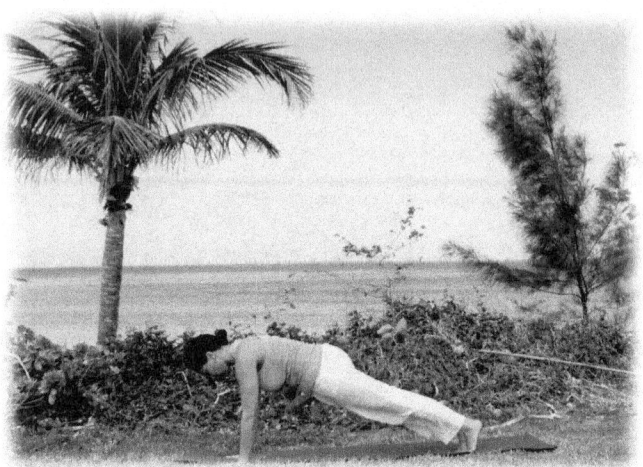

6. Exhale as you lower the knees, the chest between the hands and then the chin or forehead to the floor.

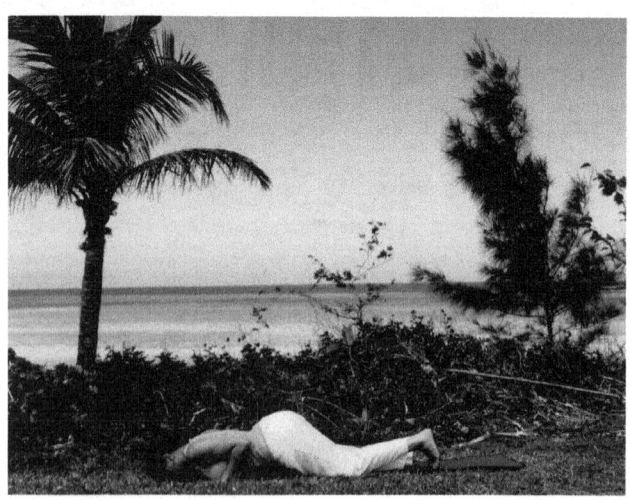

7. Inhale as you go into Cobra Pose, *Bhunjangasana*, lifting the chest, as you keep the hands under the shoulders, with the tailbone slightly tucked towards the earth. Keep the toenails on the floor.

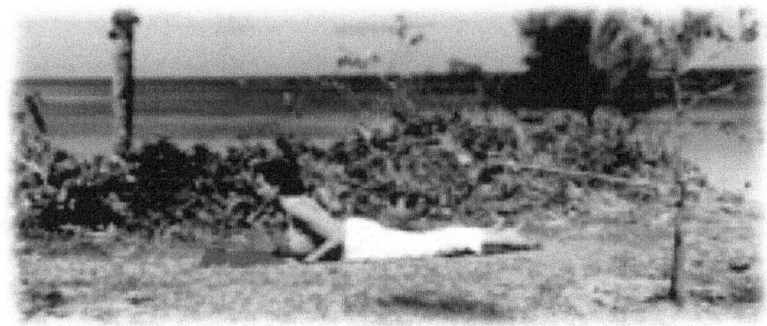

8. Exhale as you lift the hips and go into Downward Facing Dog, *Ahho Muka*

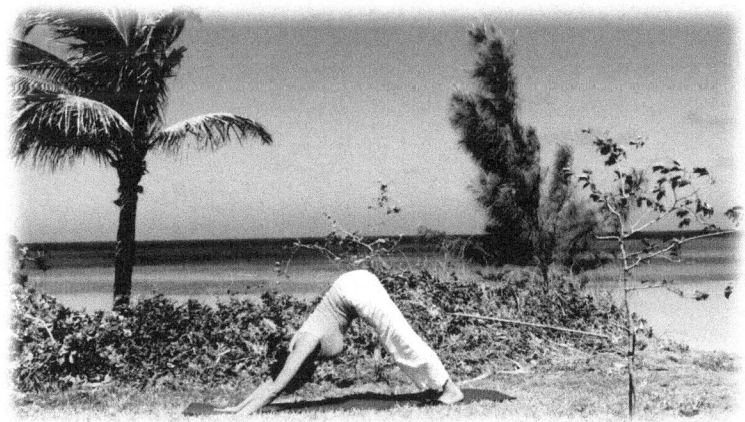

9. Inhale as you step the right foot forward into Low Lunge Pose (second side). If you foot does not get between the hands, carry it up until it does.

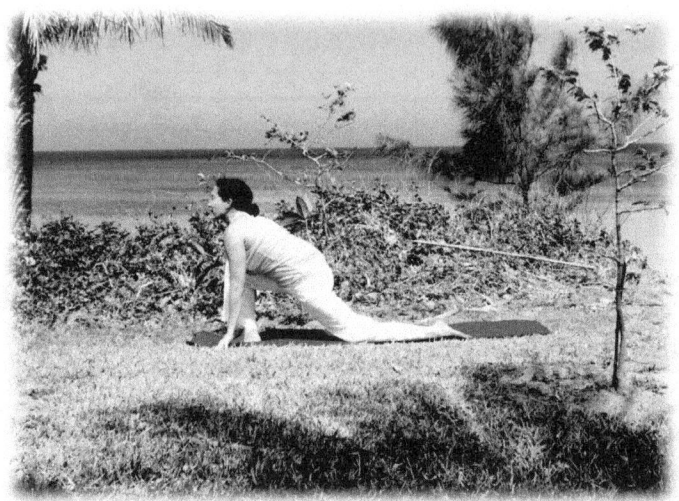

10. Exhale step the left foot forward into Forward Bend, *Uttanasana*

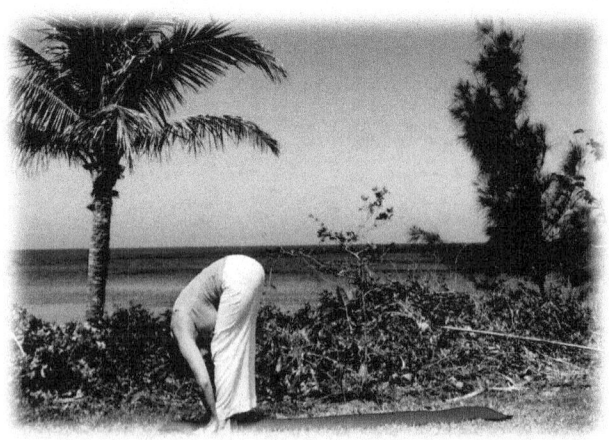

11. Inhale as you bring the hands up overhead and into a gentle backbend. Imagine you are gathering energy *(prana)* from the sun

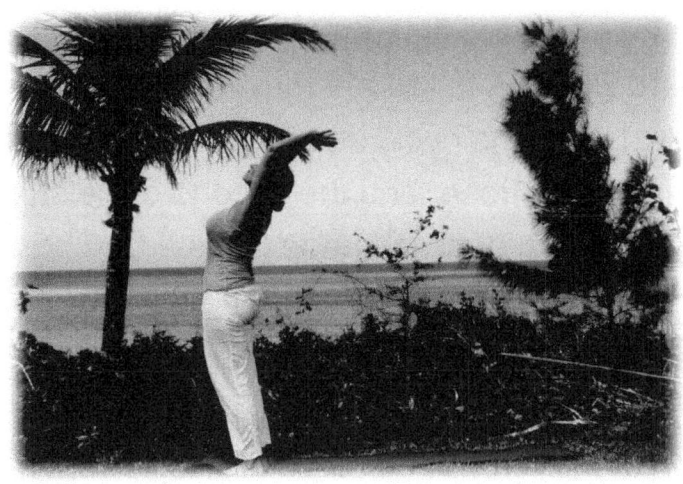

12. Exhale and bring the palms back to Prayer Pose.

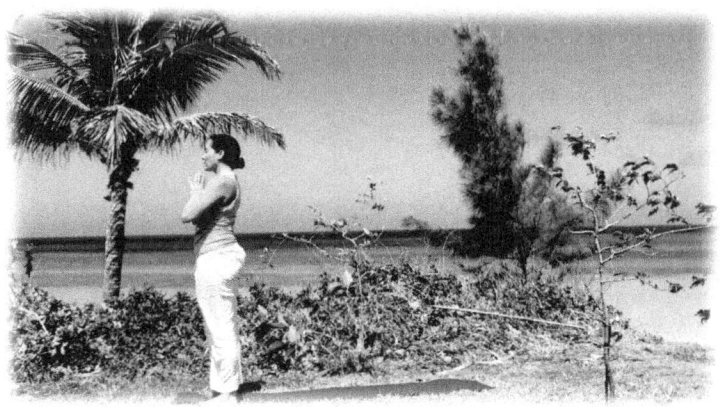

Repeat the entire Sun Salutation cycle 6-12 rounds, this time taking the left leg back into Lunge Pose. As you complete the cycle, the left leg this time steps forward first, then the right leg, in to Forward Bend. A full round may feel like two rounds, but is one cycle starting with the right leg back in Lunge Pose, and the second cycle starting with the left leg back in Lunge Pose.

Gentle Yoga Sun Salutations

-Adapted Sequence

1. Stand tall with the feet together in Mountain Pose, *Tadasana*. Bring the hands together in Prayer Pose, *Anjali Mudra* in front of the heart center. This posture is now called Equal Standing Pose. Press the feet down to the earth equally and press the hands together equally.

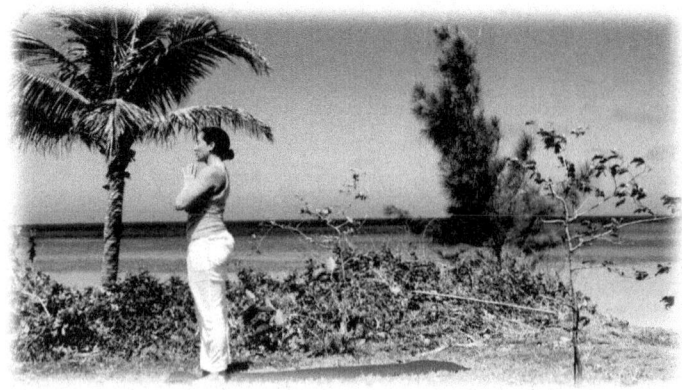

2. Inhale as you stretch the arms up overhead and slightly back, creating a backbend, only as far as comfortable (for some, this may mean not back bending, and reaching the arms overhead only.)

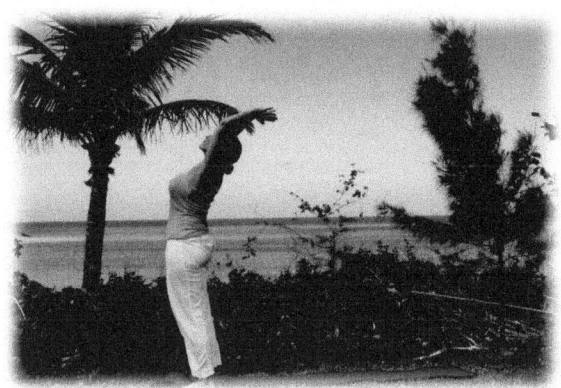

3. Exhale as you bend forward. Place the hands on the thighs or shins, extending the spine forward, or if able, touch the hands to the floor, with the hands along side the feet. Bend the knees if you need. For back injuries, keep the knees bent and the heart area lifting, extending the spine vs. forward bending fully as in the first photo on the following page.

Photos on the following page are:

(A) Half Forward Bend (for low back injuries)

(B) Full Forward Bend with the Knees Bent

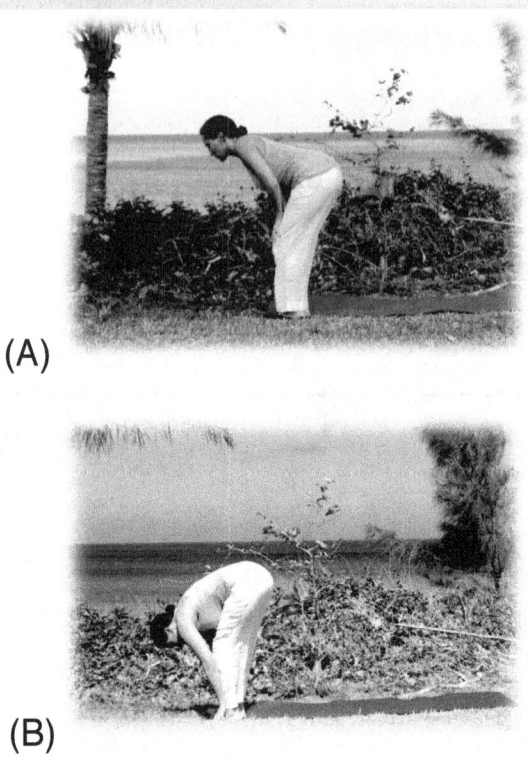

(A)

(B)

4. Inhale as you step the right leg back into Low Lunge Pose, lowering the knee to the floor.

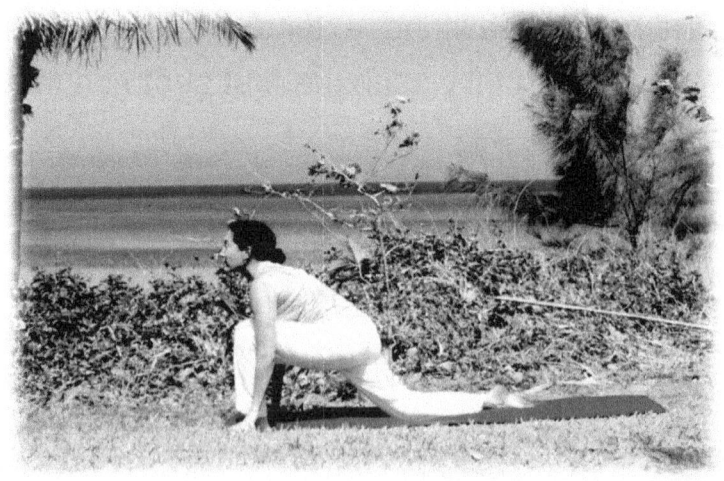

5. Step the left leg back into Table Pose, keeping the shoulders over the wrists and the hips over the knees.

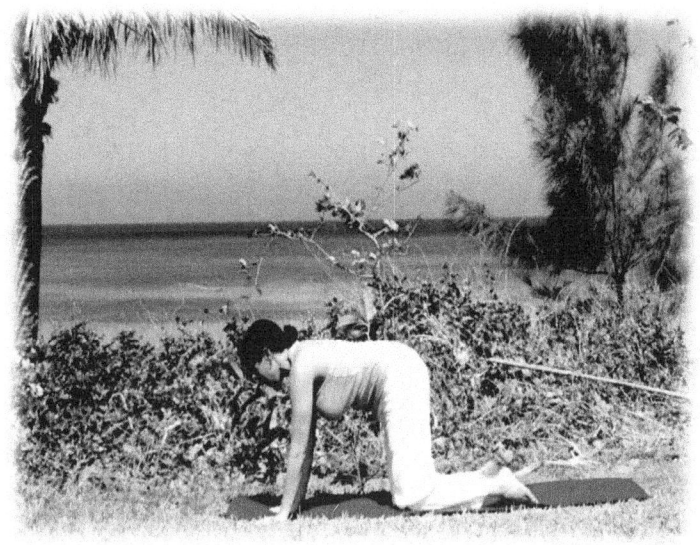

6. Inhale to Cow Pose (arch the back)

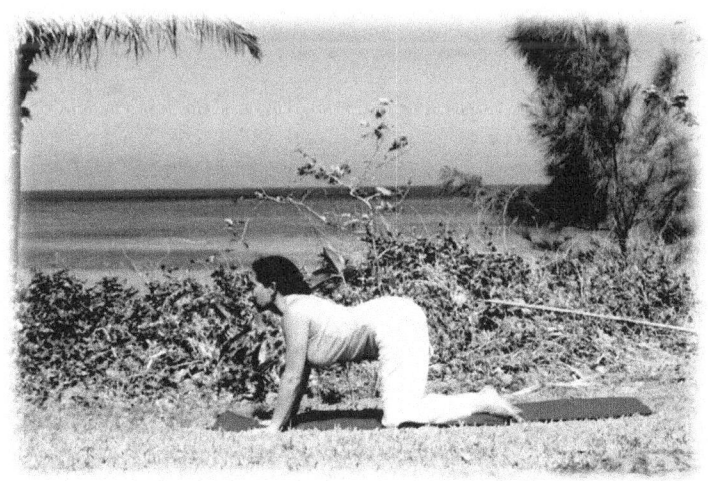

7. Exhale to Cat Pose (rounding the back).

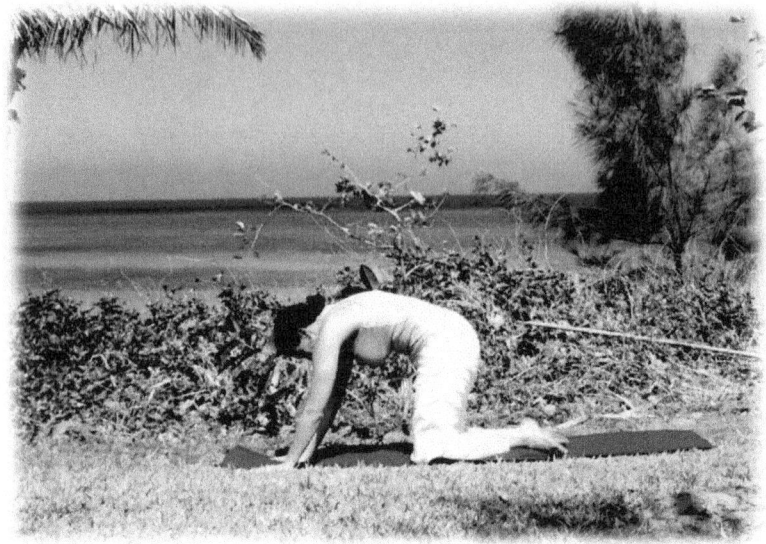

8. Inhale. Exhale into Extended Child's Pose

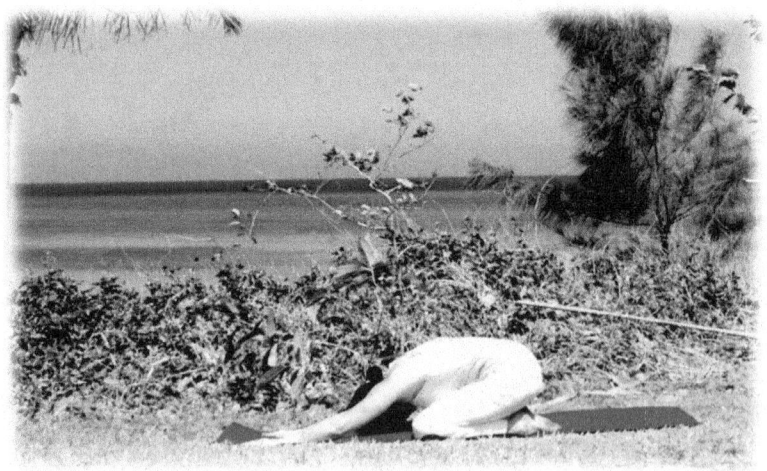

9. Inhale as you step the right foot forward into Low Lunge Pose (second side). If your foot does not get between the hands, carry it up until it does.

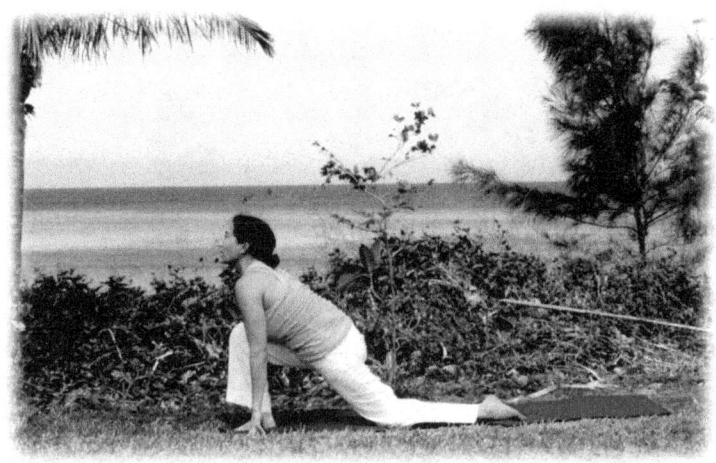

10. Exhale step the left foot forward into Forward Bend, with the hands on the legs or floor or shins as in Step 3 *(Uttanasana).*

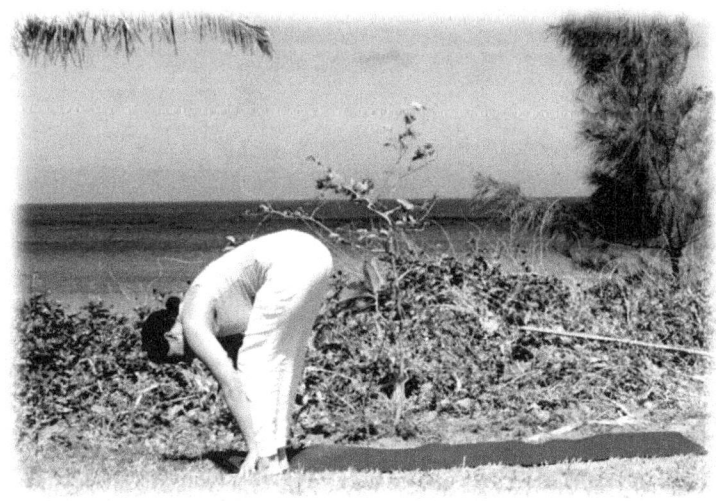

11. Inhale as you bring the hands up overhead and into a gentle backbend. Imagine you are gathering energy *(prana)* from the sun.

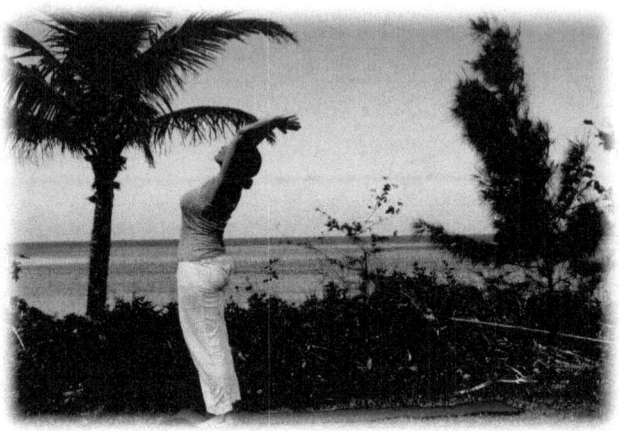

12. Exhale as you bring the palms to Prayer

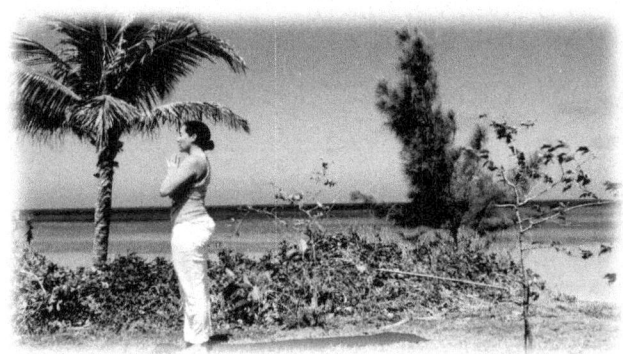

Benefits: Increases mobility, energy, flexibility, circulation and endurance, brings vitality at the beginning or middle of the day, or is calming to unwind at the end of the day. It is most powerful when done at sunrise or sunset

Standing Chair Yoga Sun Salutations

1.   Stand in Mountain Pose behind a chair. Keep the hands on the chair for balance or bring the palms in Prayer Pose.

2.   Inhale as you stretch the arms up overhead.

3.   Exhale as you bend forward, resting the head on the forearms on the chair top, the hands on the chair top or chair base.

4.   Inhale as you step one leg back to Warrior I Pose (the back foot is flat on the ground with the toes pointing 45 degrees towards the front foot). Or, go into Proud Warrior or High Lunge Pose (the back toes are curled under with the toes facing the chair). Exhale relax.

5.   Inhale one or both arms up. Exhale as you lower the arms. Switch sides or hold both arms overhead for an extra breath.

6.   Inhale as you step forward into Mountain Pose (or Downward Facing Dog). Exhale. Switch legs and inhale as you step into Warrior I, Proud Warrior or High Lunge Pose on the other side.

7.   Exhale to Mountain Pose.

8.   Inhale as you lift the heart into an upper back bend (Cobra Pose). Exhale relax.

9. Inhale as you lift the arms up. Imagine you are gathering *(prana)* energy from the sun.

10. Exhale and bring the palms back to Prayer.

Repeat 3 to 8x. See the *photos on the following pages.*

Affirmations: I am flexible. My life flows with ease. I am energized.

"My body is my temple and asanas are my prayers" -B.K.S. Iyengar

Standing Chair Yoga Sun Salutations

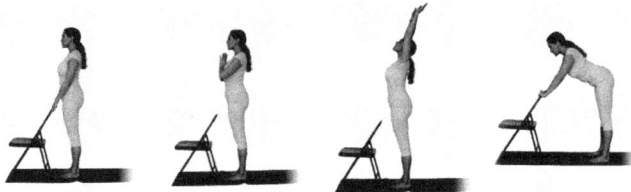

Inhale Mountain. Exhale Prayer. Inhale Arms up. Exhale Forward Bend (with the head up or resting as in the photos below).

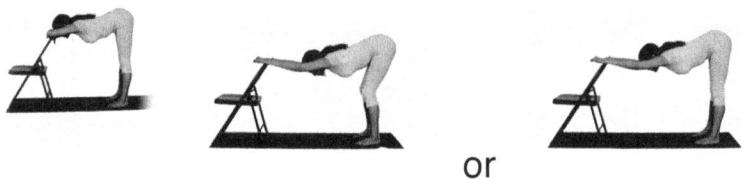

or

Forward Bend Options: The hand or head can rest on the chair top, with the knees bent or straight.

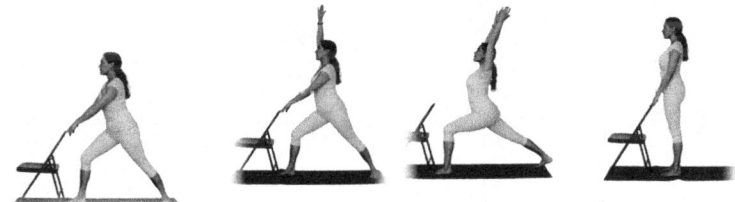

Inhale Warrior or High Lunge. Exhale relax. Inhale and lift one arm up. Exhale, lower. Inhale and lift the other arm up. Exhale, lower. Inhale and lift both arms up. Exhale, lower and step forward. Switch legs and repeat. Inhale Mountain. Exhale.

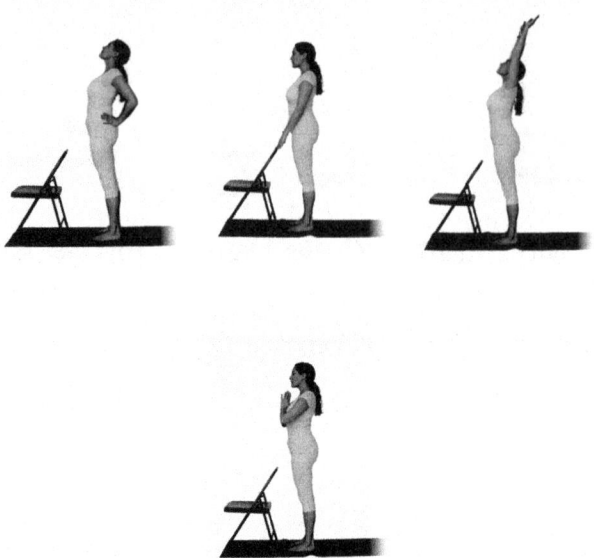

Inhale Cobra. Exhale Mountain. Inhale Arms
Up. Exhale Prayer Pose. Repeat this cycle 2-8x.

"The sun shines down, and its image
reflects in a thousand different pots filled
with water. The reflections are many, but
they are each reflecting the same sun.
Similarly, when we come to know who we
truly are, we will see ourselves in all
people." -Amma

Seated SunLight Chair Yoga Sun Salutations

1.   Bring the hands to Prayer Pose in front of the heart center.

2.   Inhale as you stretch the arms up overhead.

3.   Exhale as you bend forward.

4.   Inhale to roll the spine up, and then hold the right leg under the right knee for Lunge Pose. Exhale as you lower the leg.

5.   Inhale to lift the left knee towards the chest. Exhale as you lower the leg.

6.   Inhale Cobra Pose.

7.   Exhale relax.

8.   Inhale as you bring the hands up overhead. Imagine you are gathering energy *(prana)* from the sun.

9.   Exhale and bring the palms back to Prayer Pose.

Repeat 3 to 8x. *See photos on the next page.*

Seated Sun Salutation

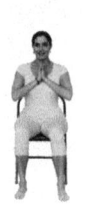 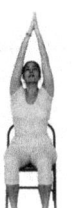 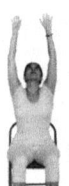

or

Prayer   Inhale Arms up

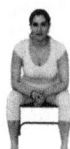 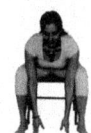 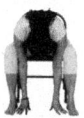

or
Exhale Forward Bend

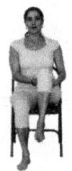 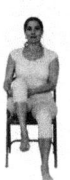

Inhale Lunge. Exhale Lower. Switch sides.

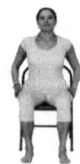 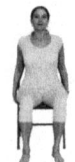 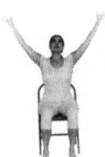 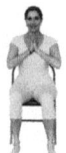

Inhale Cobra. Exhale. Inhale Arms Up.
Exhale Prayer Pose

Yoga for Everyone!

Yoga postures, called *asanas* in Sanskrit, improve flexibility, strength, and balance and calms the mind. Each pose has a different benefit. To know which benefit each pose brings, try it for yourself and experience the healing and numerous reasons to practice yoga.

Chair Yoga Hand to Foot Pose, *Hasta Padasana*

Sitting tall in a chair, lift one leg in the air and hold the leg that is stretched out. Hold the leg under the thigh, or under the calf, as comfortable, or rest the thigh on the chair base. as you stretch the leg out as in the photos below.

With Props: Place a belt or strap under the right foot. Inhale as you lift the right foot and as you extend the leg. Hold the belt with two hands, keeping the shoulders relaxed and the hands under the shoulders as in the photo below. Hold for 1-5 slow, deep breaths. Switch sides. (See the photos on the next page).

Chair Yoga Hand to Foot Pose,
Hasta Padasana

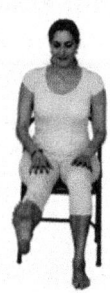 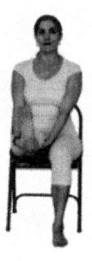

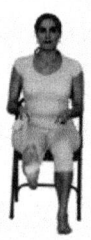

Photo (left): Leg On Chair Base
Middle photo: Holding the Leg
Photo (right): With a Belt on the Foot

Benefits: Stretches the hamstrings and legs.

Lying Down Extended Hand to Foot Pose, *Supta Hasta Padasana*

Lying on the floor, lift one leg in the air. Hold above or below the knee, or if able, hold the big toe with the index and middle fingers. Keep both feet flexed and lengthen both legs. Hold and breathe for 3-6 slow, deep breaths. Relax and breathe in this posture.

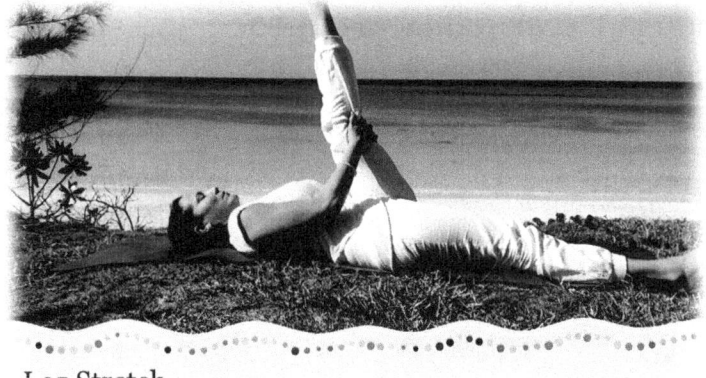

Leg Stretch

Benefits: Stretches the hamstrings, legs and calves.

Precautions: Do not overstretch. There should be neither pain nor discomfort.

Gentle Yoga Hand to Foot Pose Modification:

Lying on your back, keep the bottom leg bent with the foot on the floor, as in the photo below. Start with the knee bent as in the photo. From there, gently stretch the top leg towards the sky, as able. This is gentler for the lower back when you keep the bottom leg bent. You can also bend the leg in the air gently, as needed and still enjoy the leg stretch. From there, extend the lower leg as well for a deeper stretch. Hold for 1-5 slow, deep breaths.

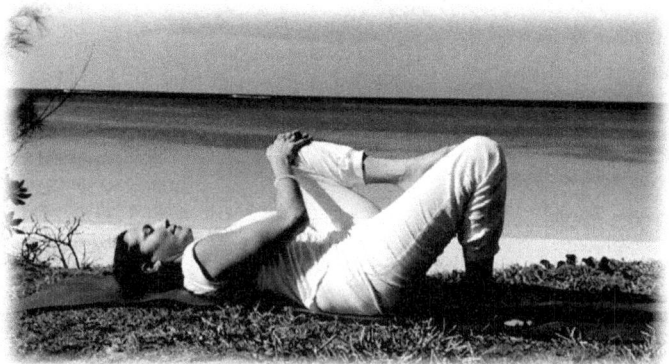

Benefits: Stretches the hamstrings, legs and calves.

Precautions: Do not overstretch. There should be neither pain nor discomfort.

Yoga for Everyone!

Standing Chair Yoga Hand to Big Toe, *Utthita Hasta Padangusthasana*

Stand facing the base of the chair. Lift one leg up and place it on the chair. Have the toes and hips pointing forward towards the chair. Inhale and stand tall as you stretch the arms overhead. Exhale as you bend forward, reaching towards the big toe. If you can't hold the left big toe with your left index and middle finger, use a yoga belt, or rest the hands on the left thigh, as shown in the second photo.

Photos below: Inhale the Arms Overhead, Exhale as you Forward Bend

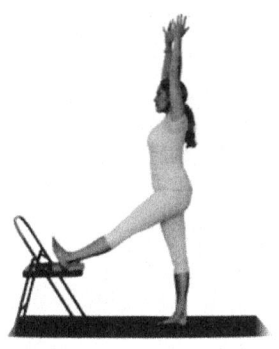 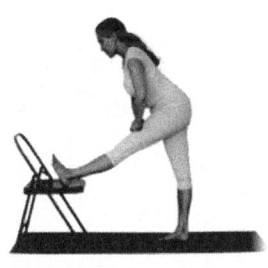

Benefits: Increases concentration, balance, leg strength and stretches the hamstrings and legs.

Staff Pose, *Dandasana*

Sitting on the floor, stretch the legs out. Place the hands by the hips. Press the hands down, into the earth, as you lift the spine tall. Flex the feet and spread the toes. Pull the toes back towards you, to engage the quadriceps (front of the thighs). Feel the whole body in the posture, strong and alert. Hold for 3-5 slow, deep breaths.

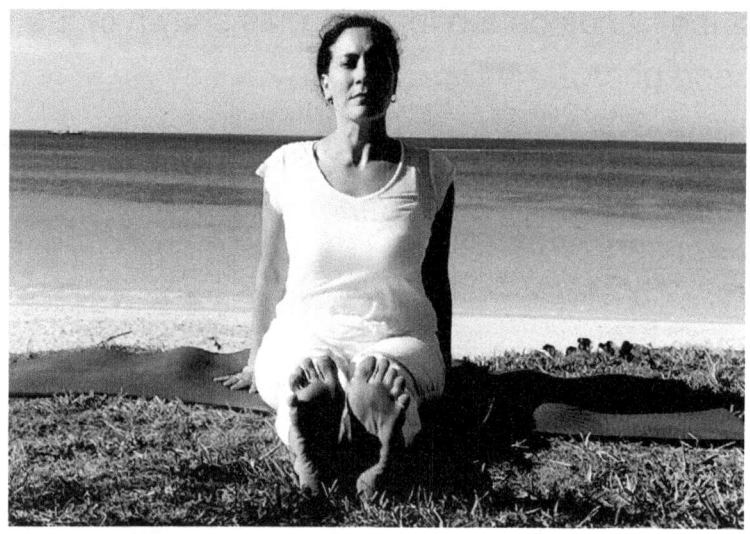

Benefits: Strengthens the back muscles and quadriceps (front of thighs) and improves posture.

Modification: Sit on a rolled blanket, cushion or towel if there is any low back pain.

Chair Yoga Staff Pose, *Dandasana*

Inhale as stretch your legs out and up. Keep the thighs on the chair base for support or rest the hands on the thighs. Hold the legs out as you take 2 to 4 slow, deep breaths. Feel the spine reaching towards the sky as the legs stretch away from the navel point (belly button area). Be mindful you don't press the back of the knees down, but instead lengthen the heels away from you.

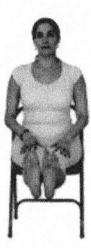

Benefits: Strengthens the back muscles and quadriceps (front of thighs) and improves posture.

Modification: For more knee support, you can practice this pose with two chairs, using a second chair in front of you to support the back of the knees and calves.

Chair Yoga Staff Pose With Props,
Dandasana

Staff Pose With a Belt

For more support in Staff Pose, wrap a yoga belt (or towel) around your feet as in the photo on the left. Hold onto the belt with your hands. As you inhale pull against the belt to sit tall, keeping the shoulders relaxed. Relax as you exhale. Place the belt under the toes. Hold one hand to each side of the belt. Inhale as you lift the legs. Keep the shoulders relaxed and the hands in line with your shoulders. Sit tall. Feel your body's strength.

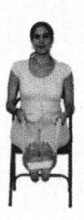

Benefits: Strengthens the back and quadriceps, stretches the legs and stretches the arms. This also strengthens the upper thigh and knee joint.

Yoga for Everyone!

Staff Pose Using Two Chairs

Using two chairs can be useful, if available. If you are in a wheelchair you can use a chair placed in front of you, as the second chair, or to support the back of the knees (The chair supporting the knees is not in the photo below). Place the feet on top of a second chair in front of you for support. Relax the hands on the thighs or stretch the arms up overhead, as in the photo below. Reach up with the fingertips and lengthen the spine as you stretch the heels away from the navel point (belly button). Try to create and "L" shape with the body.

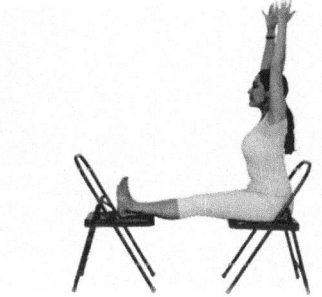

Photo: With Two Chairs

Benefits: Strengthens the back, core muscles, muscles on the thighs (quadriceps) and stretches the legs and arms.

Downward Facing Dog, *Adho Mukha Svanasana*

From Child's Pose, lift the hips off the heels, and curls the toes under. As you exhale, lift the hips in the air, creating an upside "V" shape. Keep the knees bent as needed, and try to lift the hips off the floor, to stretch the back. Think of the dogs in the pose and copy the way the dogs stretch. Hold for 1-5 slow, deep breaths.

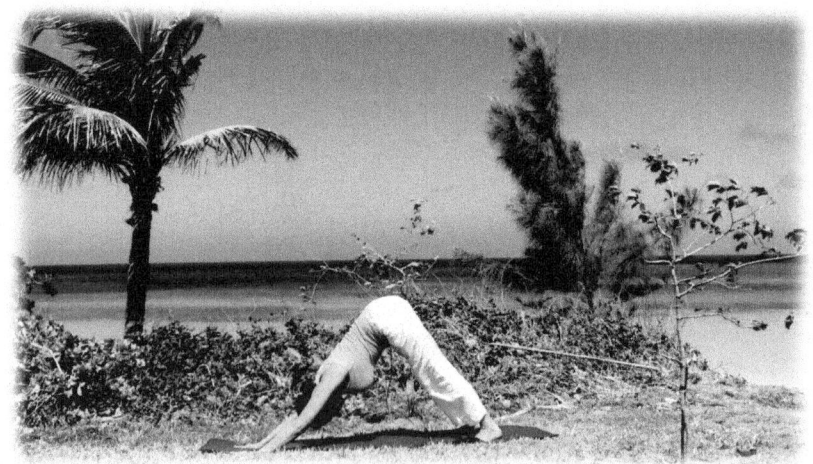

Benefits: Stretches the back and legs, and strengthens the arms. This posture also energizes the body and refreshes the mind.

Precautions: For wrist or shoulder injuries that makes it painful or unsafe to put weight on, try the Chair Yoga Downward Dog or Puppy Dog Pose.

Chair Yoga Standing Downward Facing Dog Pose, *Adho Mukha Svanasana*

Stand behind the chair. Exhale as you bend forward, placing the hands on the chair top or chair base. Walk the feet back under the feet are under the hips, creating a table like shape. If you are comfortable, try placing the hands on the chair base. Bend the knees if needed, to help the back relax. Over time the legs can straighten more.

Photo below: With the Knees Bent

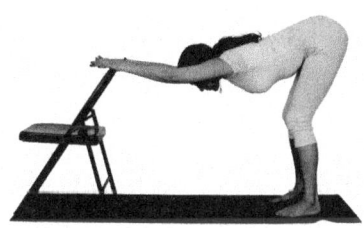

Photo below: With Hands on the Chair Base

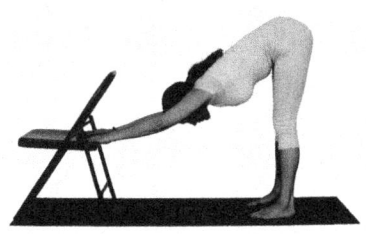

Chair Yoga Standing Downward Facing Dog Pose, *Adho Mukha Svanasana*

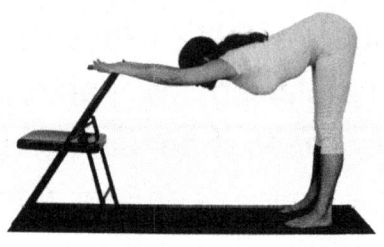

With Straight Legs

Benefits: Stretches the back and legs and calms the mind.

Precautions: If you have a low back injury or osteoporosis and are not forward bending, stand upright in Mountain Pose.

Chair Yoga Seated Downward Facing Dog, *Adho Muka Svanasana*

Inhale as you sit tall and lift the arms overhead. Exhale as you tilt the pelvis forward and reach the arms in the air. Feel the side body and spine stretching. Hold for 1-5 slow, deep breaths.

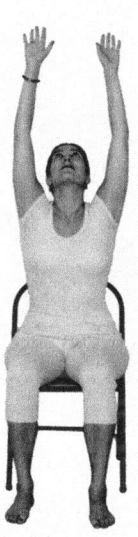

Benefits: Energizes the body. Improves circulation and relieves dullness.

Puppy Dog Pose

From Table pose (on all fours), stretch the arms and hands forward, keeping the palms facing down and the hands shoulder-width apart. As you press the hands into the earth, keep the upper arm bones lifting off the ground. Lift the tailbone reaching away from the hands, diagonally towards the sky. Think of a dog stretching here and copy the dogs.

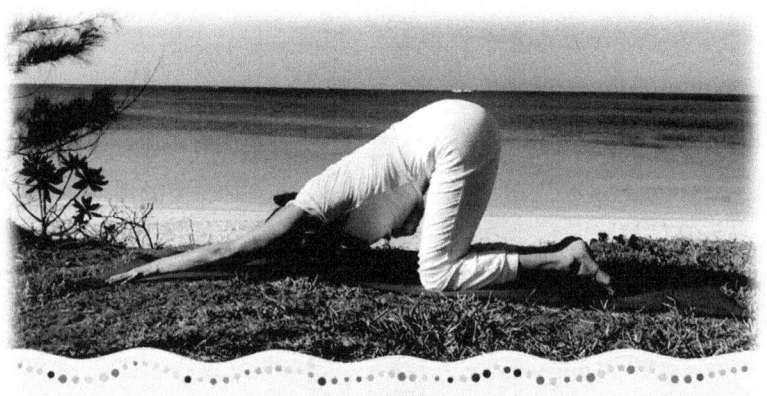

Puppy Dog Pose

Benefits: Stretches the back and sides of the body. This is a useful adaption for those with wrist or shoulder injuries, especially when Downward Dog Pose is not comfortable.

Child's Pose, *Balasana*

Sit on the heels and relax the forehead towards the earth. Resemble the shape of a fetus, curling in a ball. If it is more comfortable, rest the head on the hands under the forehead, or stretch the hands out in front of you. The big toes, knees and heels are together in this posture, but you can adapt it as needed by taking the knees apart. Hold and breathe for 2-8 rounds. This can also be a resting pose at any point during the yoga practice.

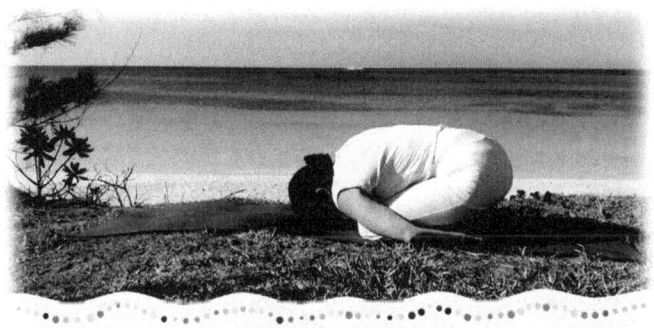
Child's Pose (Balasana)

Benefits: Restores energy, stretches the tops of the feet, calms the mind and releases the lower back and hips.

Affirmations: I have plenty of energy. I set healthy boundaries and rest when I need.

Extended Child's Pose, *Balasana*

Sit on the heels and relax the forehead towards the earth. Stretch the arms out in front of you, placing the hands shoulder-width apart. The big toes, knees and heels are together in this posture, but you can adapt it as needed by taking the knees apart. Try to push the floor forward, away from you, to release the hips and buttocks closer to the heels. Hold and breathe for 2-8 rounds. This can also be a resting pose at any point during the yoga practice.

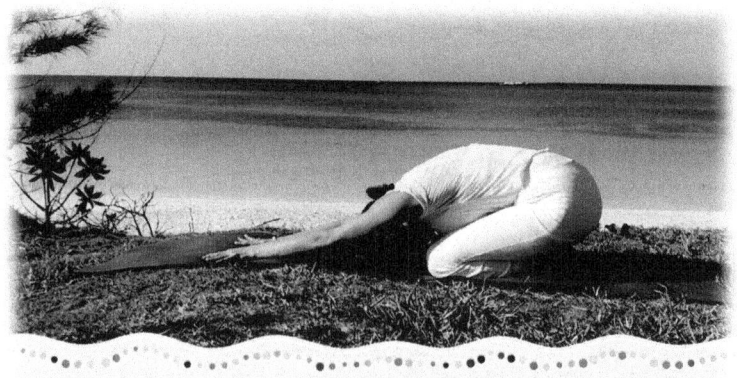
Balasana: Extended Child's Pose

Benefits: Restores energy, calms the mind, stretches the sides of the body and ankles, spine and releases the lower back and hips.

Affirmations: I reach my full potential. I relax into the unknown.

Upside Down Child's Pose

If Child's Pose is not comfortable, due to knee or ankle discomfort, you can practice the posture upside down instead. Lie on your back and hug the knees into the chest. Hold for 3-5 slow, deep breaths.

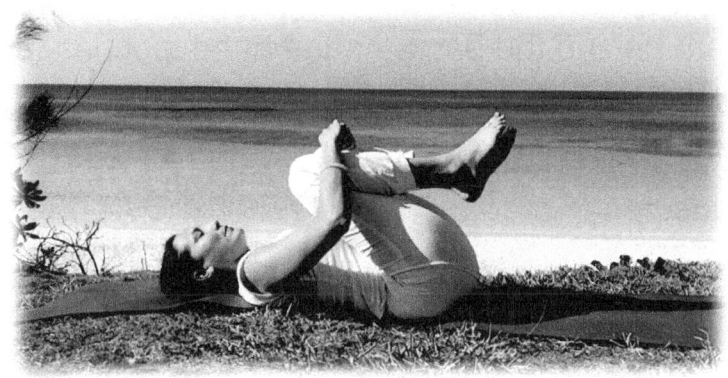

Benefits: Restores energy, calms the mind and releases the lower back and hips.

Affirmations: I have plenty of energy. I set healthy boundaries and rest when I need. I relax and feel at ease.

Child's Pose Shoulder Variation,
Balasana

Sit on the heels and relax the forehead towards the earth. The big toes, knees and heels are together in this posture, but you can adapt it as needed by taking the knees apart. Interlock the fingers behind the back. As the head touches the earth, stretch the hands back and up overhead, as in the photo below. Hold and breathe for 2-4 rounds.

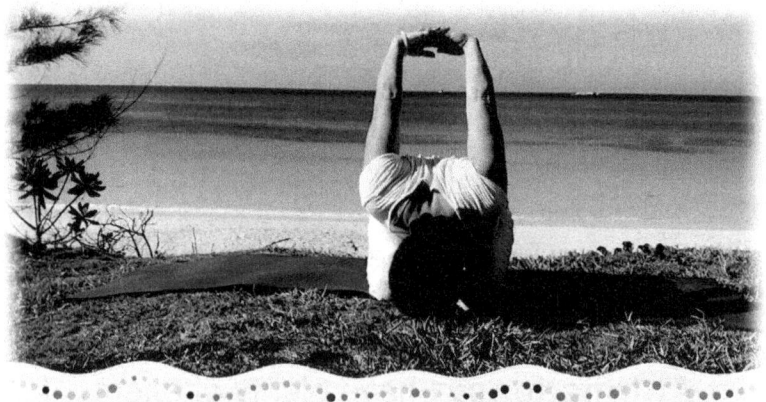

Child's Pose Shoulder Variation: interlock the fingers behind you.

Benefits: Releases shoulder and upper back tension and increase mobility in the shoulder joints. This pose also stretches the ankles.

Lunge Pose, *Anjaneyasana*

From Downward Facing Dog Pose or Table Pose, step one foot between the hands. Slide the back foot back, as much as able, keeping the hands on the ground. As you inhale try to lengthen the spine and lift the heart area. Release the back thigh forward. Hold for 1-5 slow, deep breaths. Switch sides.

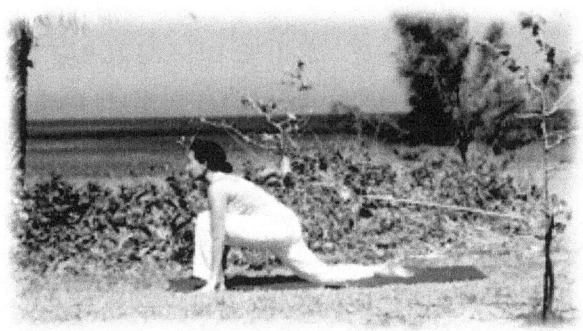

Gentle Yoga Lunge Modifications

Repeat the steps as above, but use yoga blocks below each hand, for more support. You can also place a towel or blanket under the back knee for more cushioning to the knee joint. Hold for 2 breaths each side and build up to 5 breaths each side, over time. There should be neither strain in the body nor pain in the joints.

Benefits: Stretches the front of the thighs and opens the hips.

Wide Lunge Pose/Lizard Pose,
Utthan Pristhasana

From Downward Facing Dog Pose or Table Pose, step the left foot forward and place it to the left of the left hand, on the left side of edge of the yoga mat. Slide the right foot back, as much as able, keeping the hands on the ground. As you inhale try to lengthen the spine and lift the heart area. Exhale as you relax the chest towards the earth. Release the right thigh forward. Hold for 1-5 slow, deep breaths. Switch sides.

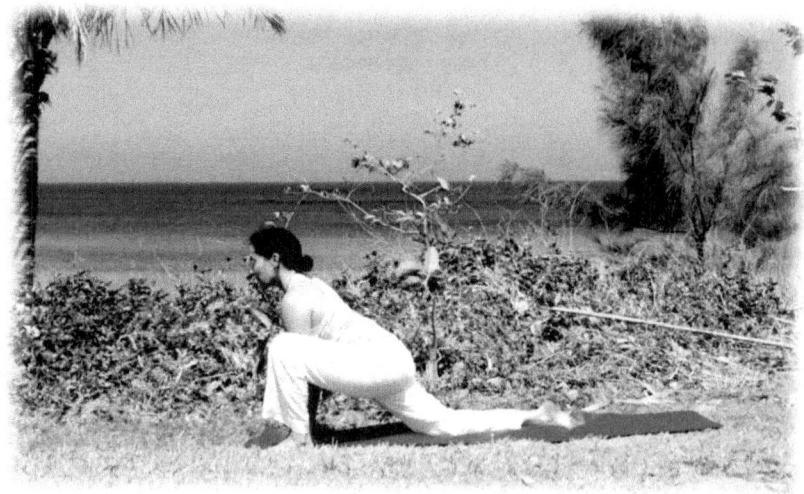

Benefits: Stretches the front of the thighs, quadriceps and hip flexors.

Chair Yoga Low Lunge, *Anjaneyasana*

Sitting tall, hold the right thigh under the right knee, as you lift the navel towards the leg. Keep the shoulders relaxed and lift through the core. Hold for a few slow, deep breaths. Exhale as you lower the leg. Switch sides.

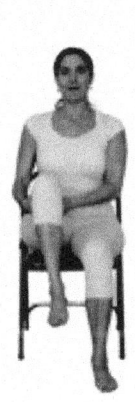

Benefits: Eases sciatic joint and low back pain, prevents sciatica and increases mobility.

High Lunge Pose/Horse Rider's
Pose, *Ashva Sanchalanasana*

Sit facing the right side of the chair with your right waist facing the back of the chair. Place the right thigh fully on the chair, and release all or part of the left buttocks off the chair. Keep your right hand on the chair back for support and balance assistance. If you are able and comfortable, extend the left leg back into High Lunge Pose.

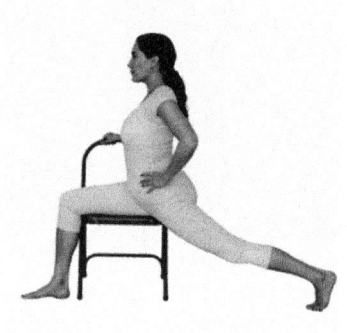

Benefits: Strengthens the legs, assists with balance and opens the hips.

Seated High Lunge Pose Arm Variation, *Ashva Sanchalanasana*

From High Lunge Pose (see previous page) inhale as you lift your left arm up. Hold and breathe for 1 to 5 slow, deep, rhythmic breaths. Switch sides. **Seated Proud Warrior:** If able and comfortable, try lifting both arms up.

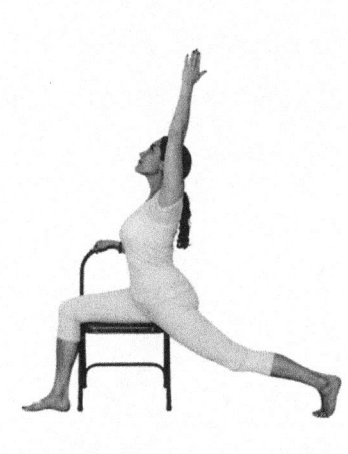

Benefits: Strengthens the legs, tones the arms, increases stamina, balance and concentration and opens the hips.

Affirmations: I am courageous. I am strong.

Standing Supported High Lunge/ Horse Rider's Pose, *Ashva Sanchalanasana*

From the Standing Warrior 1 Pose (see the Standing Sun Salutations), come into High Lunge Pose by curling the back toes under, so that the toes are facing forward towards the chair. You can also come into this posture from Standing Chair Yoga Downward Facing Dog. From Downward Facing Dog step one foot forward and lift the heart and head. Switch sides.

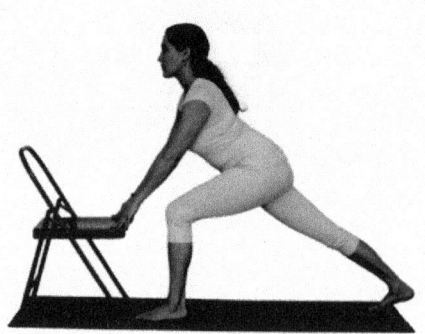

Benefits: Strengthens the legs, stretches the back calf muscle and opens the hips.

Affirmations: I am powerful. I am strong.

Standing High Lunge Pose/Horse Rider's Pose, *"Proud Warrior"*,

Ashva Sanchalanasana

Stand behind the chair. Step your right foot back 3 to 4 feet. Have the back toes curled under, facing the chair. Hold on to the chair back for support, or, if able, inhale as you lift one or both arms overhead. Repeat 2 to 5x or hold steady for 2 to 5 slow, deep breaths.

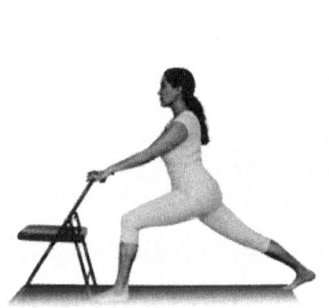 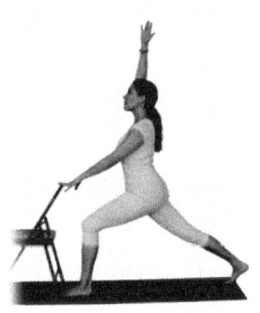

Photo above left: With Support

Photo right: One Arm Up

Benefits: Strengthens the legs, stretches the back calf muscle and opens the hips.

Affirmations: I am powerful. I am strong.

Standing High Lunge Pose/Horse Rider's Pose, *"Proud Warrior"*,

Ashva Sanchalanasana

Photo: Proud Warrior Pose with Both Arms Up.

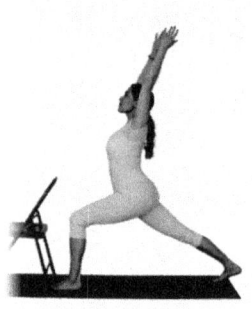

Benefits: This pose increases mobility of the hip joint and can ease hip and low back pain. With the arms overhead it strengthens the heart and tones the arms and side waist.

Precautions: For knee injuries or balance concerns, try the standing or Seated Lunge Pose. You can also place the back knee on the floor if able, with the hands on the chair base. Place the back knee on a blanket for more comfort (Low Lunge Pose).

Affirmations: I am powerful. I love my life.

Yoga for Everyone!

Reflections

Take a moment to pause and notice the areas in your life where you are already strong and centered, like a peaceful warrior. Are there other areas that you can bring more confidence, strength and balance to?

"There is something good in all seeming failures. You are not to see that now. Time will reveal it. Be patient." Swami Sivananda

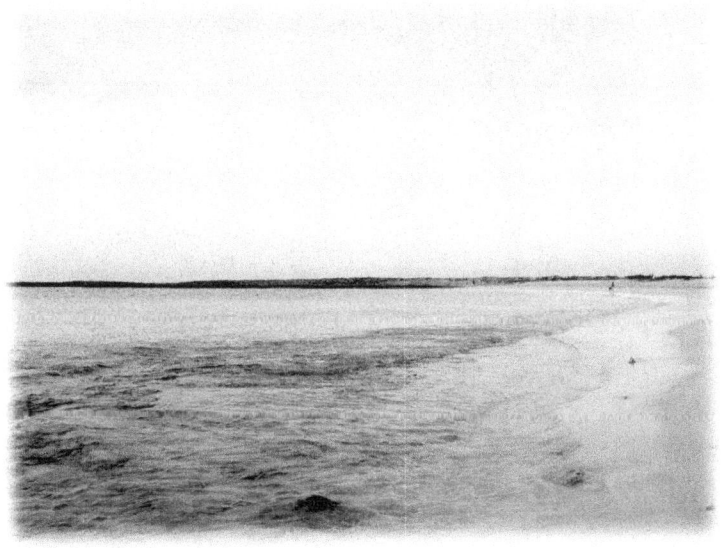

Powerful or Fierce Pose, *Utkatasana*

Stand tall in Mountain Pose. As you exhale lower the hips, as if you are about to sit in a chair. Keep the toes facing forward and the knees facing the toes. Stretch the arms out in front of you, and eventually overhead. If able, bring the upper arms by the ears with the palms facing each other. Hold for 1-5 slow, deep breaths.

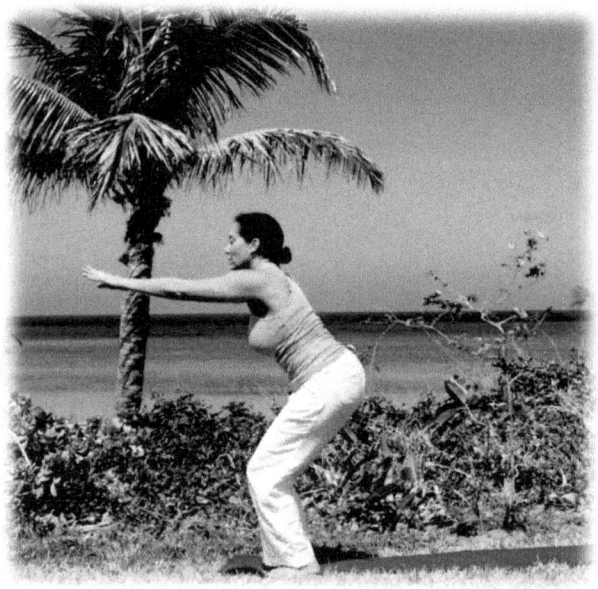

Benefits: Strengthens the legs, tones the arms and improves balance.

Affirmations: I am strong and centered. I am powerful and peaceful.

Yoga for Everyone!

Chair Yoga Powerful Pose (Seated to Standing)

Press the hands into the chair arms or chair base and lift your body up and down. Have the toes pointing forward and keep the knees facing the toes (trying not to let the knees move towards each other). Repeat 5x. Inhale as you lift and exhale as you lower. Hold the posture with the hands on the hips or reach them overhead for 2 to 5 slow, deep breaths.

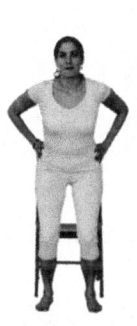 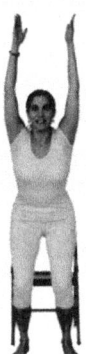

Photo left: Hands on Hips

Photo right: Hands Overhead

Benefits: This is called the Powerful Pose in Sanskrit (commonly called the Chair Pose), because it brings great strength to the body (and mind). It strengthens the legs, arms and core. This pose can help prevent falls and keeps the body strong to get up and down from chairs, bed, baths and walkers. It also aids general movements.

Precautions: For shoulder discomfort, keep the hands on the hips. For knee discomfort, remain seated and lift the arms only.

Standing Powerful Pose, *Utkatasana*

Stand behind the chair. Hold on to the chair back with the feet hip-width apart and the toes pointing forward with the knees facing the toes. Exhale as you bend the knees. Try not to let the knees collapse in towards each other. Hold the body in this posture for 2 to 3 deep breaths, or go in and out 3 to 5x. Keep the shoulders relaxed.

If able, lift one hand at a time (or both hands) off the chair and hold for 1 to 3 slow, deep breaths. Switch sides. See the photos on the following page.

Chair Yoga Standing Powerful Pose,
Utkatasana

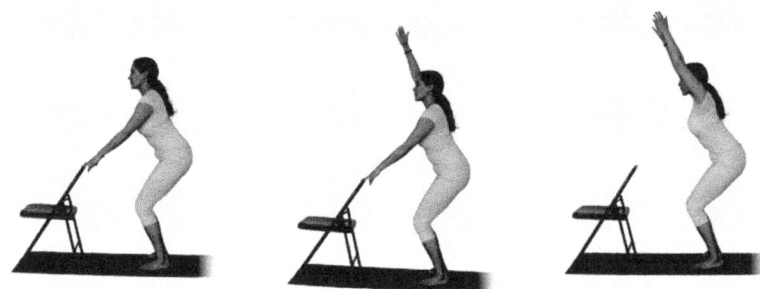

Photo Top Left: Hands on the Chair
Photo Top Right: One Hand Up
Bottom Photo: Both Hands Up

Benefits: Strengthens the legs, tones the arms, stretches the side body and helps tone the waist. The standing version helps strengthen the legs and promotes an increased awareness and sense of balance (physically and mentally).

Chair Yoga Seated Powerful Pose

Raise the arms overhead as you sit tall in the chair. Hold for 5 slow, deep breaths, feeling your strength (outer and inner strength).

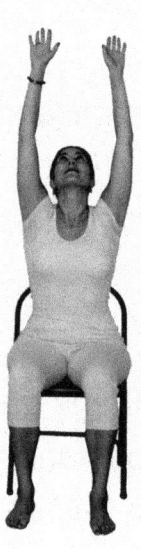

Benefits: Tones the arms, stretches the side body and energizes the body and mind.

"Windmill Pose"/Revolved Standing Wide-Legged Forward Bend,
Paravritta Prasarita Padottanasana

Stand with your feet wider than hip-width apart and the toes pointing forward. Inhale, stand tall and lift the heart. Exhale and fold forward, resting the hands on floor (or on a yoga block). Only go as far as comfortable and bend the knees if needed. Place your right hand on the floor and gently twist the spine to the left. Stretch the left arm skyward. Keep the head centered. If comfortable, gently look up towards the sky over the left shoulder. Hold as long as comfortable. Switch sides.

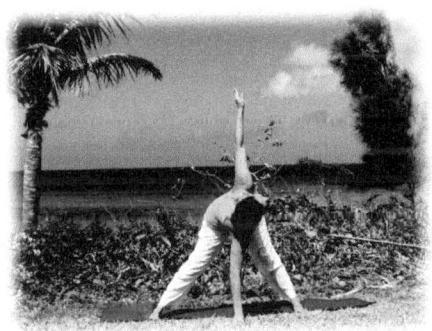

Benefits: Stretches and strengthens the legs, aids digestions and improves flexibility in the spine. Spinal twists also calm the nerves.

Precautions: Do not bend and twist if you are pregnant, have osteoporosis or back injuries.

Chair Yoga Revolved Standing F "Windmill Pose", *Paravritta Prasarita Padottanasana*

Stand with your feet wider than hip-width apart and the toes pointing forward. Inhale, stand tall and lift the heart. Exhale and fold forward, resting the hands on a second chair top, base or lower chair bars. Only go as far as comfortable. Place your left hand on the left hip and gently twist the spine to the left. Keep the head centered or, if comfortable, gently look up towards the sky over the left shoulder. Hold as long as comfortable. Switch sides.

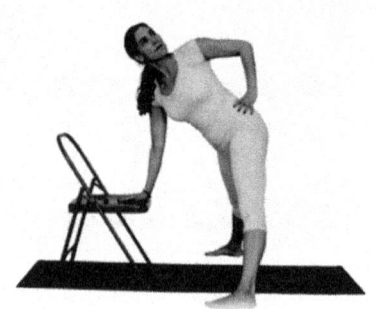

Benefits: Stretches and strengthens the back and legs, decreases back pain, increases awareness in the feet, opens the hips and is calming. Spinal twists can also ease and balance the digestive system.

Precautions: Bend the knees and keep the spine upright for back pain or injuries that are aggravated by this pose. If you are pregnant, twist from above the upper ribs only.

Chair Yoga Seated Windmill Pose

Place the feet hip width apart. Inhale as you sit tall. Exhale as you fold at the hips into a forward bend resting the forearms on the thighs as pictured below. Keep your buttocks on the chair base.

Step 1: Forward Bend with the Arms on Thighs

Step 2: Gently Twist the right from the forward bend, looking over the right shoulder. Make sure there is no discomfort in the neck. Repeat to the left. Hold each side for 2-5 slow, deep breaths.

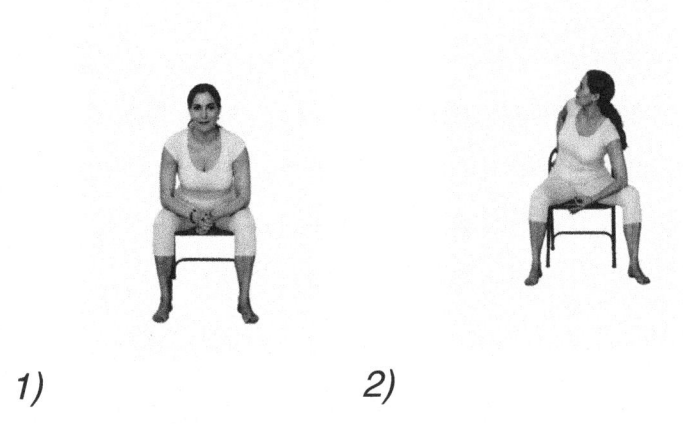

1)   2)

Step 3: If comfortable, release one hand to the floor. Relax and breathe.

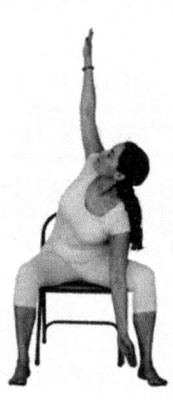

Benefits: Decreases back pain and improves flexibility in the spine and back. Spinal twists can also ease and balance the digestive system.

Precautions: Keep your head centered if you have vertigo or experience dizziness. Do not twist if there are any conditions or injuries that are aggravated by this pose. If you are pregnant, twist from above the upper ribs only.

Forward Bends

Forward Bends are calming for the mind and bring flexibility to the spine. There are many ways to practice forward bends, including from standing positions, seated on the floor or standing or seated using a chair for support.

For lower back injuries, osteoporosis or other conditions that cause pain or are contraindicated for forward bending, sit tall instead and focus on the breath. Modify by practicing Mountain Pose, *Tadasana* instead. For general low back comfort, some find it gentler to bend the knees in the forward bends. Make sure that there is no strain and never back pain in the posture (or in any yoga posture). Use the breath to relax in the pose.

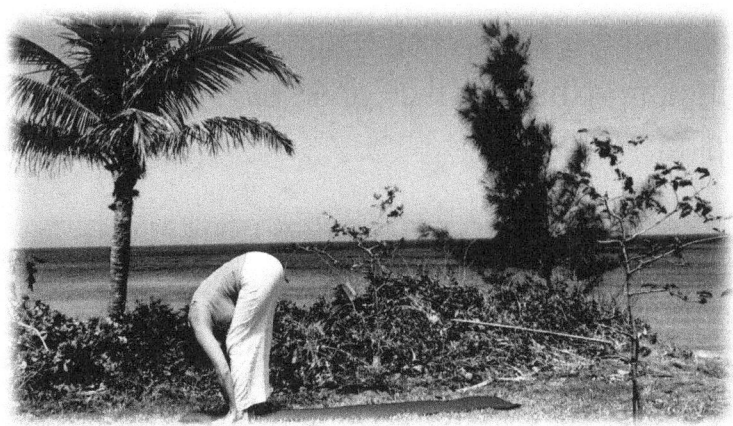

Standing Forward Bend, *Uttanasana*

From a standing Mountain Pose, bend the knees and gently fold forward as you exhale. Allow the spine to lengthen towards the earth, and relax the neck. Place the hands on the floor, or the thighs or shins for lower back comfort, if needed (see the following page). Over time, the legs can straighten.

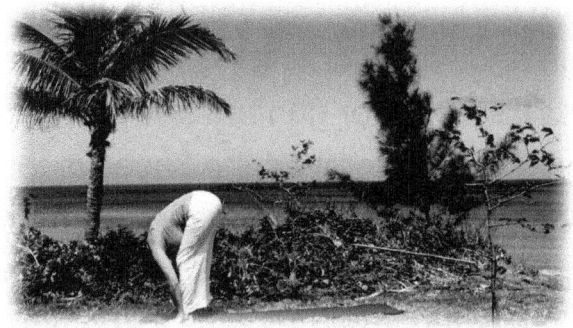

Benefits: Stretches the back and legs (hamstrings and calves), soothes the nervous system, relaxes the neck and spine and is calming.

Precautions: Do not forward bend if you have osteoporosis, disc or low back injuries. In some cases you can modify by bending the knees and lifting the chest (see next page).

Affirmations: I relax and let go of negativity.

Standing Gentle Forward Bends

Half Way Lift in a Forward Bend

From a standing Mountain Pose, bend the knees and gently fold forward as you exhale. Keep the spine lengthening and place the hands on the thighs or shins. Keep the heart area lifting and the spine lengthening. Feel a gentle arch (backbend) to the pelvic area, as you tilt the pelvis slightly forward and then lengthen the spine (opposite action of rounding the back). Over time, the legs can stretch straight. The exact position of the pelvis and back will vary, based on comfort and prior injuries.

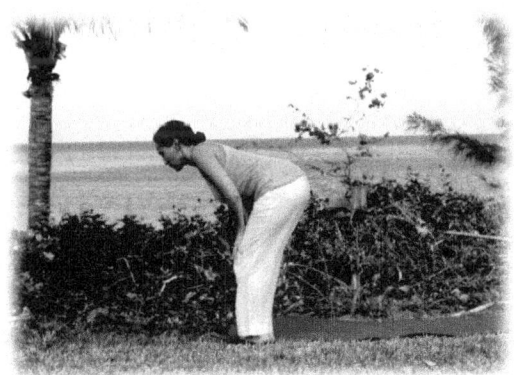

Benefits: Stretches the back, increases flexibility and mobility in the hip joint, gently stretches the legs and is calming.

"Rag Doll Pose"

From a standing Mountain Pose, bend the knees and gently fold forward as you exhale. Hold each hand to the opposite elbow. Feel the spine relax completely, like a rag doll. If it feels good on your body, you can also gently sway a few times from side to side, while holding the elbows. Relax the neck and jaw and let go of all tension.

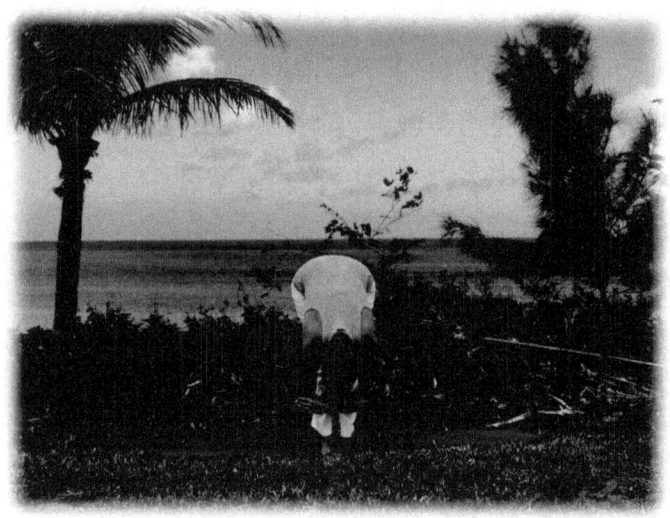

Benefits: Stretches the back, strengthens the thighs and knees, reduces stress, anxiety and depression and relieves tension in the back, neck and spine.

Affirmations: I let go and surrender.

Seated Forward Bend,
Paschimottanasana

Sit on the floor with your legs stretched out. Inhale deeply. Exhale and hinge forward at the hips, placing the hands on the legs, or holding the big toes with the index and middle fingers. Make sure there is no strain behind the knees or in the lower back. If it is comfortable, exhale and relax the chest towards the legs, releasing the head down. **With props**: Place a yoga belt around the feet, under the toes and hold the sides of the yoga belt. Pull against the belt to help lengthen the spine.

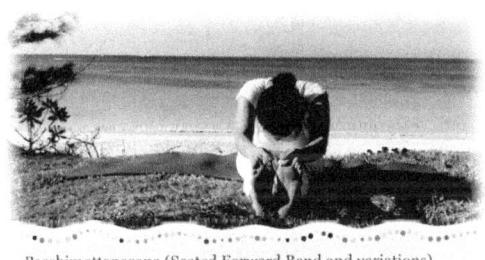

Paschimottanasana (Seated Forward Bend and variations)

Benefits: Stretches the back and the legs and calms the mind.

Precautions: Do not practice this pose if you have a slip disc, osteoporosis, sciatica or a back condition.

Affirmations: I relax. I surrender and let go.

Gentle Seated Forward Bend, Half Way Lift, *Paschimottanasana*

Sit on the floor with your legs stretched out. Inhale deeply. Exhale and hinge forward at the hips, placing the hands on the legs, or holding the big toes with the index and middle fingers. Bend the knees if needed, and make sure there is no strain behind the knees or in the lower back. Inhale, lift and lengthen the spine. Exhale, relax.

Half Way Lift with Knees Bent

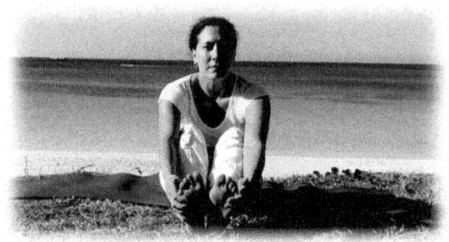

Half Way Lift with Straight Legs

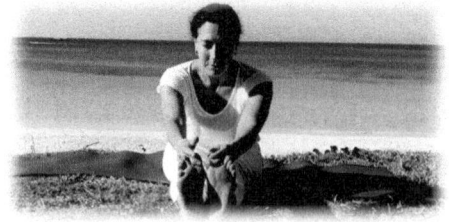

Benefits: Stretches the back and the legs, shoulders and hamstrings, improves digestion, soothes headaches, reduces fatigue and calms the mind and nervous system.

Yoga for Everyone!

Gentle Seated Forward Bend With the Knees Bent, *Paschimottanasana*

Sit on the floor with your legs stretched out. Inhale deeply. Exhale and hinge forward at the hips, placing the hands on the legs, or holding the big toes with the index and middle fingers. Bend the knees to make sure there is no strain behind the knees or in the lower back. As you inhale, lift and lengthen the spine. Exhale and relax the chest towards the legs. Hold for 3-5 slow, deep breaths.

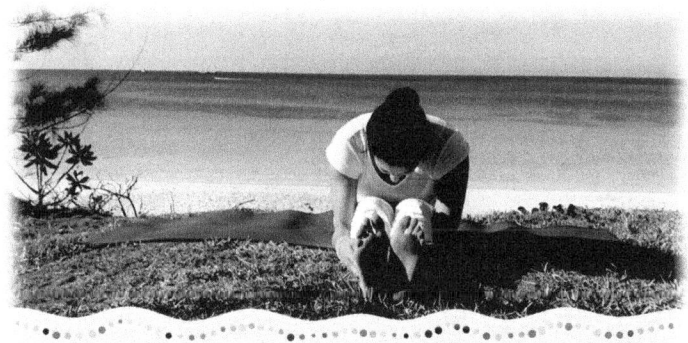

Paschimottanasana (West Side Stretch or Forward Bend)

Benefits: Stretches the back, improves digestion, soothes headaches, reduces fatigue and calms the mind and nervous system.

Affirmations: I relax. I surrender and let go.

Seated Chair Yoga Forward Bend

Inhale as you sit tall. Exhale as you bend forward. Rest the arms on the thighs or touch the ground, as able and comfortable. You can take the legs hip width apart or wider, or whichever is the most comfortable. You can also choose to keep the head and chest lifted (as in the second photo below).

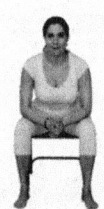 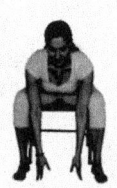 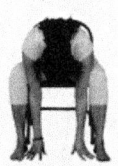

Benefits: Increases flexibility of the back and hips and is calming for the mind.

Precautions: If you have a slip disc, sciatic, low back injury or osteoporosis and are not forward bending, sit up right in Mountain Pose.

Affirmations: I am flexible. I let go with ease.

Wide-Legged Forward Bend

Stand with your feet farther than hip-width apart and the toes pointing forward. Inhale, stand tall and lift the heart. Exhale and fold forward, resting the hands the outer legs, ankles, or holding the big toes with the index and middle fingers. Relax the neck and hold for 3-5 slow, deep breaths. If there is any strain in the hamstrings, bend the knees slightly.

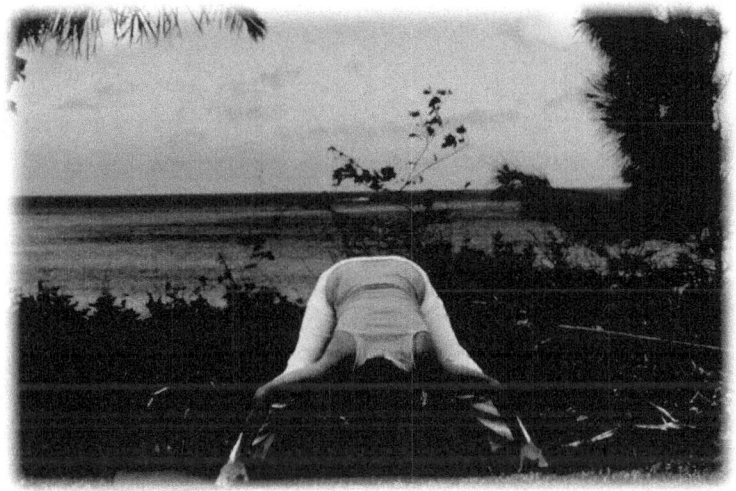

Benefits: Stretches the hamstrings, legs and relaxes the back.

Standing Chair Yoga Wide-Legged Forward Bend, *Prasarita Padottanasana*

Stand with your feet farther than hip-width apart and the toes pointing forward. Inhale, stand tall and lift the heart. Exhale and fold forward, resting the hands on a second chair top, chair base or to the chair bars.

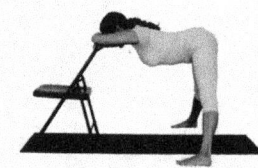 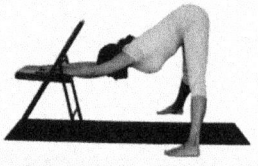

Photo (left): Head on the Forearms
Photo (right): Hands on the Chair
Photo below: Hands on the Chair Lower Legs

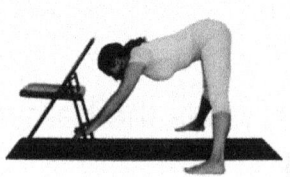

Benefits: Stretches and strengthens the back and legs, brings awareness in the feet, opens the hips and is calming.

Yoga for Everyone!

Wide-Legged Forward Bend

Precautions: Keep your head up for vertigo, or blood pressure issues. Bend the knees and/or keep the spine upright if there is any lower back pain. Bend the knees softly if you need, to ease any strain in the hamstrings or behind the knees. If you have osteoporosis or a lower back injury, stand tall instead of forward bending.

Chair Yoga Seated Wide-Legged Forward Bend

Separate the feet wider than hip-width apart, or as wide as is comfortable. Keep your buttocks on the chair base. Inhale as you sit tall. Exhale as you fold at the hips into a forward bend. Reach the hands towards the earth (see the photo on the next page). You can also place your forearms on the thighs as in the photo below, as comfortable, or place the hands on a yoga block on the floor or on a second chair in front of you. Hold for 1-5 slow, deep breaths. See the photos on the following page.

Chair Yoga Seated Wide -Legged Forward Bend

Photo (left): Forward Bend with Arms on Thighs
Photo (right): Hands to the Floor with the Head and Spine Lengthening

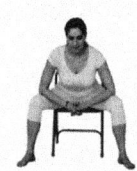 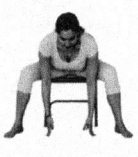

Benefits: Relaxes the back, gives flexibility to the hips and spine, and is calming.

Precautions: Do not practice forward bends if you have osteoporosis, low back or disc injuries. Keep your head up for vertigo, dizziness or blood pressure issues.

Affirmations: I relax. I let go. I surrender. I trust the flow of life.

Seated Chair Yoga Extended Leg Forward Bend, *Paschimotanasa*

Hold on to the chair back or base. Stretch the legs out, and pull the toes towards the face. Exhale as you bend forward from the hips, keeping the buttocks evenly pressing into the chair base. Keep the sternum (chest bone) lifting and the spine lengthening. If comfortable, exhale as you bend forward.

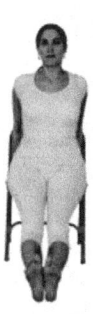

Precautions: Bend the knees softly if you need, to ease any strain in the hamstrings or behind the knees. If you have osteoporosis or a lower back injury, sit tall and breathe instead of forward bending.

Seated Forward Bend With Two Chairs, *Paschimottanasana*

With two chairs, place the feet up on a second chair (you can also support the back of knees on the second chair base, not pictured in photo). Inhale as you sit tall. As you exhale, reach towards the toes (or use a belt wrapped around the feet). Lift the sternum (chest bone) to create length to the spine (avoid collapsing the upper back or pressing the back of the knees down). Hold for 1 to 5 slow, deep breaths.

Photos below: Inhale, Arms Up. Exhale Fold

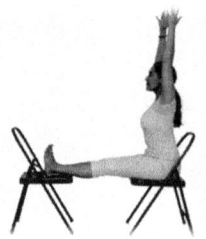 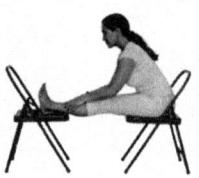

Seated Forward Bend With Two Chairs

Benefits: Stretches the back and legs and calms the mind.

Precautions: Do not forward bend if you have low back injuries, osteoporosis, or if there is any pain or discomfort.

Yoga for Everyone!

Chair Yoga Bound Angle Pose
Forward Bend, *Baddha Konasana*

Sit tall in a chair. Lift one foot up at a time onto a second chair placed in front of you. Bring the feet together. Relax the knees out to the sides. Keep your buttocks on the chair base. Inhale as you sit tall. Exhale as you fold at the hips into a forward bend. Rest the arms on the thighs, or if able, hold on to the ankles or toes. Inhale, extend and lengthen the spine. Exhale as you fold forward. Hold for 1 to 5 deep breaths.

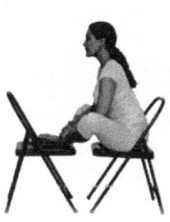

Benefits: Improves flexibility in the inner thighs, groins and the knees and prepares the body for a meditation pose. This pose can ease prenatal and menstrual discomfort.

Precautions: Keep your head up for vertigo, dizziness or blood pressure issues. Keep the spine upright (not bending forward) for lower back pain or related injuries.

One-Legged Pigeon Pose Forward Bend Variation, *Eka Pada Kapotasana*

From Table Pose (on all fours), place one knee between the hands as you stretch the other leg back. Inhale and lengthen the spine, staying upright or fold forward and rest the forehead on the hands, as able. If comfortable, reach the arms and hands forward as in the variation shown in the photo below. Relax the hips towards the earth and press all five toenails on the back foot into the earth. Hold and breathe for 1-8 slow, deep breaths.

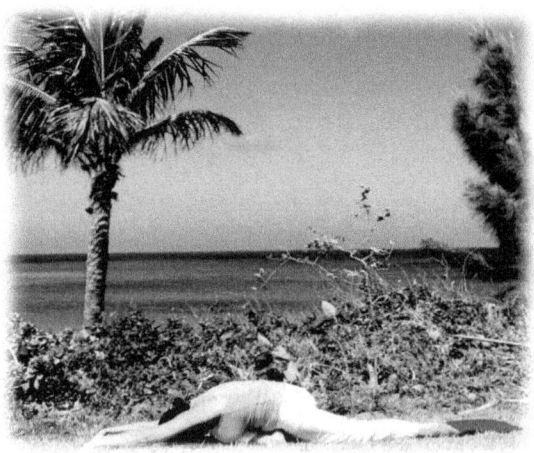

Benefits: Stretches the gluteus muscles, the groins and psoas and relaxes the back. This pose is useful for those sitting long hours at a desk.

Old Sage Pose (Standing Pigeon Pose)

From Mountain Pose, place the feet hip width apart, with the toes pointing forward. Lower the hips towards the earth as you place the left ankle on the right thigh. Flex the left foot and spread the toes. Hold for 1-5 slow, deep breaths.

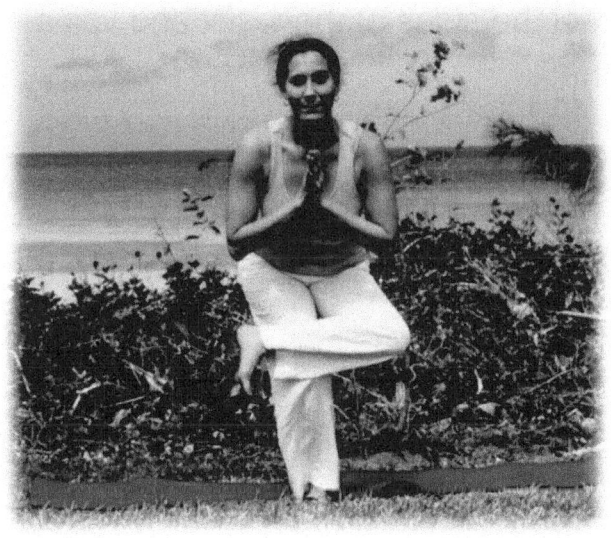

Benefits: Strengthens the legs, stretches the gluteus, groins and psoas.

Precautions: for knee injuries, try the Seated Pigeon Pose. Make sure there is no pain or strain in any of the joints.

Affirmations: I am wise. I trust my inner knowing. All I seek is within.

Chair Yoga One-Legged Pigeon Pose
Forward Bend, *Eka Pada Kapotasana*

Sit with the feet hip width apart. Place your right foot on top of your left thigh. Exhale as you bend forward. Keep the sternum (chest bone) lifting and the buttocks releasing into the chair base. Feel the sides of the waist and spine lengthen.

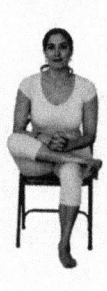

Benefits: Increases the range of motion externally in the hip socket and opens the hips flexors, stretches the gluteus, groins and psoas. This seated version is useful to practice at the desk or while on long flights to stretch the hips and legs.

Triangle Pose, *Trikonasana*

Stand with the feet 3-4 feet apart and balance the weight equally on both feet. Turn the right toes to the left 45 degrees and the left toes to the left. Stretch the arms out in a "T" shape. Inhale deeply and as you exhale, shift the hips to the right as your stretch the spine to the left. Lower the left hand to the left thigh, shin or floor (behind the left ankle). Stretch the right hand up creating a "T" like shape with the arms. Hold for 1-5 slow, deep breaths. Switch sides.

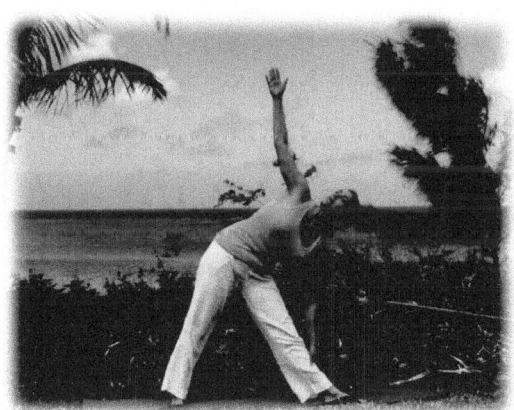

Benefits: Stretches the spine, legs hips and lower back, strengthens the legs, knees, ankles and abdominals and improves balance.

Standing Chair Yoga Triangle Pose,
Trikonasana

Stand behind the chair. Step your left leg 3 to 4 feet back. Turn your left toes towards the chair (spiral the thighbone inward). Turn the body so that your torso faces to the left. Place the right hand on the top of the chair or chair base (as in the photos below). Inhale. Exhale as you shift your hips to the left and place your left hand on the hip (or stretch your left arm towards the sky). Twist the spine and torso gently to the left (towards the sky). Hold for 3 to 5 deep breaths per side, or inhale to come out and exhale to go into the posture, repeating 3x.

Photo: With Hands on the Hip and Chair Top

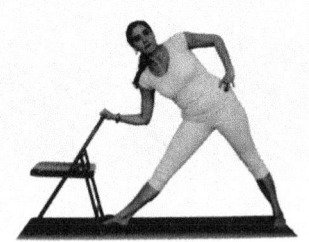

Benefits: Stretches the spine, legs, calves, hamstrings, ankle joints, hips and lower back. Increases leg strength and balance.

Photo (below left): Triangle Pose With the Hand on the Chair Base

Photo (below right): Triangle Pose With the Top Arm Extended

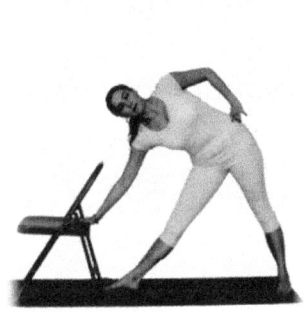 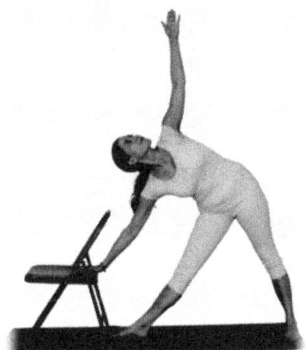

Benefits: Stretches the sides of the body, legs, groin muscles, hamstrings, claves, chest and spine, strengthens the legs, knees and oblique muscles.

Seated Chair Yoga Triangle Pose,
Trikonasana

Inhale as you stretch your arms away from the heart in a "T" shape. Exhale as you lean to one side. Inhale as you bring the torso back to the center. Exhale as you lean to the other side. If comfortable, when leaning to the right, gently turn the head and spine, twisting from the right ribs towards the left ribs (skywards). Gaze at the left fingers. Repeat 3x or hold for 3 to 5 breaths.

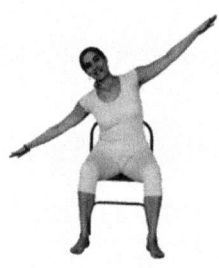

Benefits: Stretches the sides of the body and the arms. Flexibility is improved by bending the spine sideways. This posture also helps the mind to focus inward (on the heart area).

Seated Triangle Pose Variation,
Trikonasana

Follow the steps on the previous page for the Triangle Pose. Extend the right leg out to the right and flex the foot. Exhale as you lean to the right with the arms extended. Hold for 1 to 3 slow breaths. Switch sides.

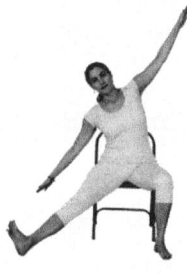

Photo: Triangle Pose With the Leg Extended

Benefits: Stretches the sides of the body, the arms and the extended leg. Flexibility is improved by bending the spine sideways. This posture also helps the mind to focus inward (on the heart area).

Extended Triangle Pose,
Utthita Trikonasana

Stand with the feet 3-4 feet apart and balance on both feet. Turn the right toes to the left 45 degrees and the left toes to the left. Stretch the arms out in a "T" shape. Inhale deeply. As you exhale shift the hips to the right as your stretch the spine the left. Lower the left hand to the left leg or floor (behind the left ankle), and stretch the right hand up and over the left ear. As you do this press both feet into the earth. Hold for 1-5 slow, deep breathes. Switch sides.

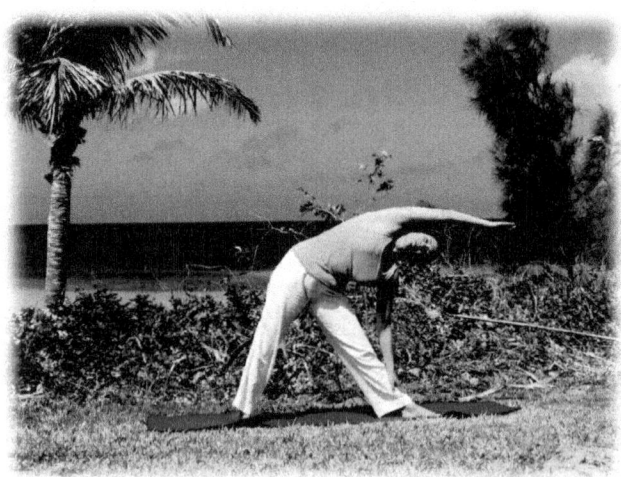

Benefits: Stretches the spine, hips and lower back. Increases leg strength and balance.

Seated Extended Side Angle Pose,
Utthita Parsvakonasana

Rest your right thigh on the chair base. Stretch the left leg out to the left, with the toes turned in slightly towards the chair. Stretch the arms away from the heart in a lateral "T" shape. Inhale as you sit tall. Exhale, lean to the right, resting your right arm on the right thigh, or the right hand on the floor behind the right foot. Stretch the left arm along side the ear (or place it on the left hip). Gaze at the left upper arm. Hold for 1 to 3 deep breaths. Switch sides.

Photo below: Extended Side Angle Pose with the arm on the Thigh

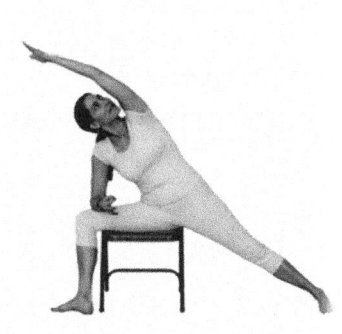

Photo below: Extended Side Angle Pose with the Hand on the Floor

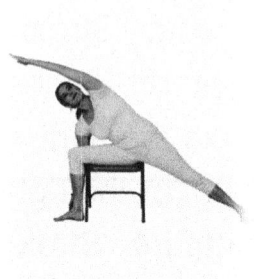

Deepening Alignment: To increase the hip opening, gently guide your right thigh back so that the knee moves towards the little toe side of the right foot. While the thigh moves back, the spine twists gently towards the sky (right ribs moving towards the left ribs or sky).

Benefits: Stretches the sides of the body, groin muscles, calves and spine, legs and opens the hips.

Precautions: For shoulder discomfort, place the top hand on the top the hip. For neck discomfort keep the head looking forward or down.

Affirmations I am flexible. I am strong. I am energized.

Standing Chair Yoga Crescent Moon Pose, *Chandrasana*

Stand tall with the feet hip-width apart and the toes pointing towards the chair or turn your body (legs and feet included) to the side with your right waist facing the chair back. Place the right hand on the chair top for support. Balance the weight on both feet as evenly as you can. Inhale your left arm up, and lean to the right, keeping the weight even on the feet. Switch sides. If able, release both hands off the chair top, and try the posture as you balance. For a deeper stretch through the lower back, keep more weight on the left foot as the left arm reaches up. Reverse for the right side (put more weight on the right foot as the right arm is up).

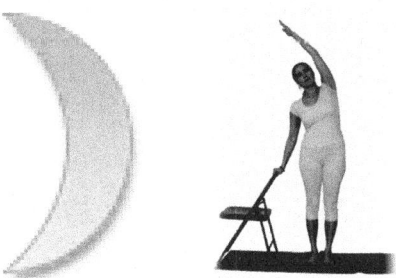

Benefits: Stretches the side body, improving flexibility of the spine and improves balance.

Seated Crescent Moon Pose,
Chandrasana

Sit tall with the head centered over the spine. Inhale as you lift the left arm up and curve the spine to the right, in a crescent shape. You can also bring the palms together, or interlock the fingers overhead, as in the second photo. Press the buttocks into the chair base evenly as you lean to the side. Hold for 1-5 slow, deep breaths. Switch sides.

Arms Apart   *Fingers Interlocked*

Benefits: Stretches the spine and stretches and tones the waist. Since this posture stretches the side waist and the muscles by the ribcage, it can also allow for more ease with breathing. It also improves concentration.

Seated Crescent Moon Pose with a Belt, *Chandrasana*

With Props: Pull the belt apart overhead with your hands as you curve the spine to one side. For arm resistance, pull the belt apart strongly while you keep the shoulders relaxed. Hold for 1-5 slow, deep breaths. Switch sides.

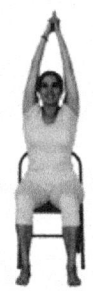 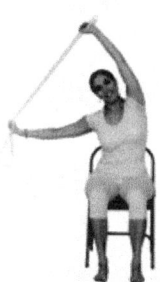

Photo on Left: Center Position
Photo on Right: With a Belt

Benefits: Stretches the spine and stretches and tones the waist. Since this posture stretches the side waist and the muscles by the ribcage, it can also allow for more ease with breathing.

Affirmations: I flow in life with ease.

Reflections

Take a moment to pause and reflect on how you are already flexible in your life. How does that feel? Which areas of your life (physically, mentally or emotionally) can you be more flexible in?

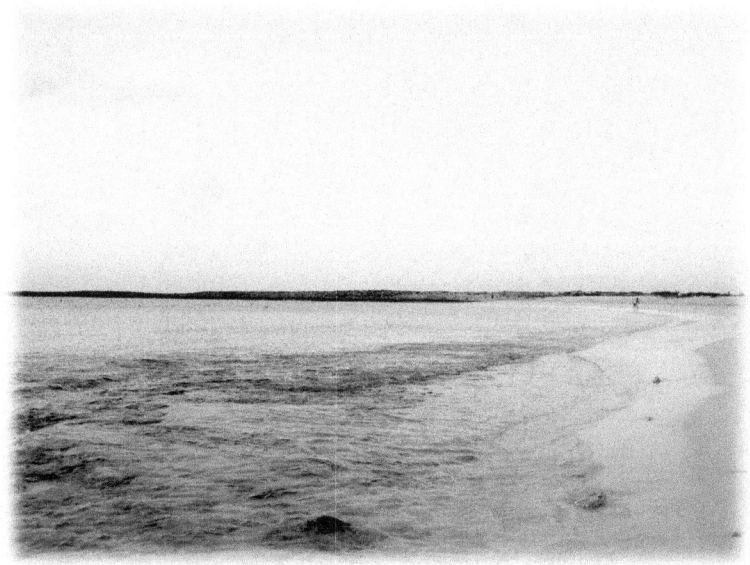

"You cannot do yoga. Yoga is your natural state. What you can do are yoga exercises, which may reveal to you where you are resisting your natural state." – Sharon Gannon

Standing Chair Yoga Tree Pose, *Vrksasana*

Stand to the left side of the chair. Hold your right hand on the chair. Place the left heel behind the left ankle, shifting the weight to the right leg and foot. Focus the eyes and mind on one stationary point in front of you. Hold the posture and take 5 deep breaths.

Photo: Standing Tree Pose, Heel Behind the Ankle

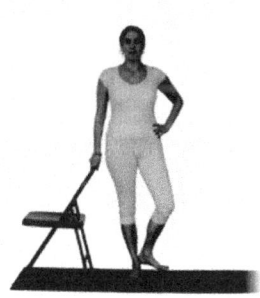

Benefits: Improves balance (physically and emotionally) and concentration, strengthens the legs, ankles and stretches the thighs and groins.

From Tree Pose, place the foot that is behind

the ankle to the inside of the opposite shin. Keep the eyes and mind focused on one point. Extend the outer arm to the side or on a diagonal away from the body. Hold for 1 to 5 slow, deep breaths. Switch sides.

Photo: Standing Tree Pose, Foot on the Lower Leg and the Arm Extended

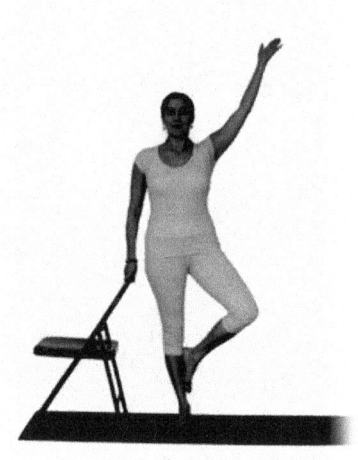

Benefits: Improves balance, concentration and helps prevent falls by bringing awareness to the weight shifts on the feet. The tree symbolizes life and increased vitality.

Tree Pose (next steps)

From Tree Pose (previous photos), carry the foot that is inside of the opposite shin higher up, towards the inside of the inner thigh, as high as you can comfortably go. Balance and breathe. Focus the eyes on one point. Relax the shoulders, stomach and face. Feel the crown (top) of the head lifting up towards the sky as the standing leg and foot root themselves into the earth. Hold for 1 to 5 deep breaths. Switch sides.

From either the seated or standing Tree Poses (see previous pages), lift one arm up as you inhale. Exhale as you lower the arm. Switch sides. Repeat 2x. Then lift both arms up overhead and focus the eyes on one point. Breathe and balance for as long as you are comfortable. Keep the shoulders, face and stomach relaxed. Stretch the sides of the body and feel the standing leg and foot rooting into the earth. Switch sides. Come out of the pose to rest. See the photos on the following page.

Seated Chair Yoga Tree Pose,

Vrksasana

Seated: Bring the palms to Prayer Pose. Inhale as you lift your arms up overhead in a "Y" shape or with the palms together (see the photo on the following page). Bring one heel behind the opposite ankle with the toes on floor. Then try to lift your toes on that same foot you placed behind the ankle. Focus the eyes on one point in front of you. Hold and balance for 3 to 5 deep breaths. Switch sides. Or inhale as you go into the pose and exhale as you release. Repeat 3x. For a gentle variation rest the hands on the thighs, as below.

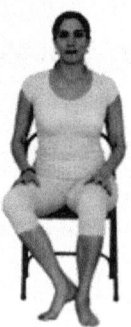

Seated Tree Pose with the Foot in the Inner Ankle

Seated Chair Yoga Tree Pose,
Vrksasana

Photo: Seated Tree Pose with the Foot in the Inner Ankle and the Arms Extended

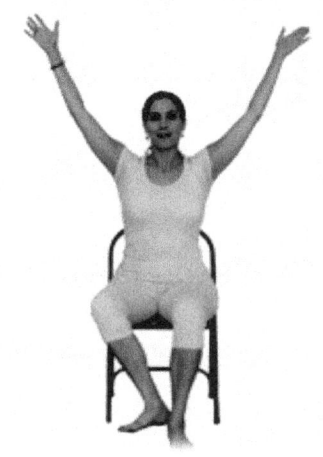

Benefits: Improves concentration and flexibility in the hips and stretches the thighs and groins. The tree symbolizes life and increased vitality.

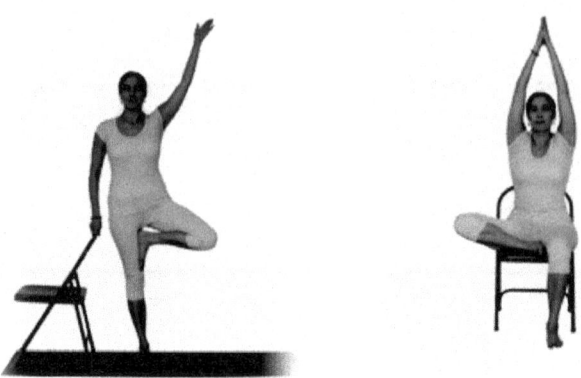

Photo (top): Standing Tree (Foot on Inner Thigh)

Photo (bottom): Seated Tree With Foot on the Chair Base and the Arms Up

Benefits: Improves balance, concentration and confidence, stretches the spine and waist and brings awareness to the weight shifts on the feet, which can help prevent falls. The tree symbolizes life so can increase your vitality and energy.

Affirmations: I am balanced. I am energized. I feel my vitality with each breath. I am grounded and relaxed.

Warrior III, *Virabhadrasana III*

From Mountain Pose (standing tall with the feet together), step one foot back and lift the back leg up as you stretch the foot back, creating a "T" like shape with the body. The arms reach forward as you stretch the leg back, finding balance. Focus on one point on front of you or on the floor that is not moving. Hold and breathe for 1 to 5 deep breaths. Switch sides.

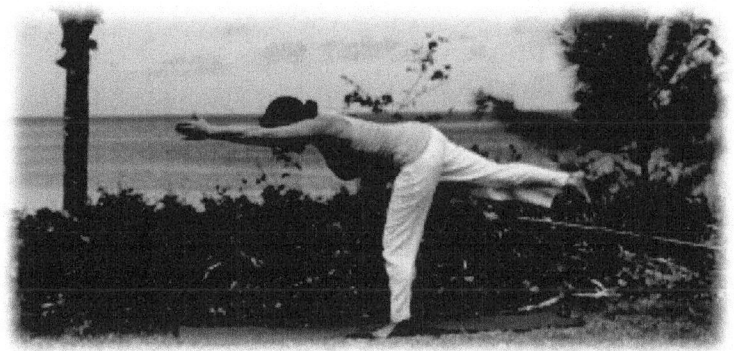

Benefits: Improves balance, stability and concentration, strengthens the legs and stretches the arms, legs, and torso.

Affirmations: I am brave. I am strong. I am balanced.

Chair Yoga Standing Warrior III,
Virabhadrasana III

From Table Pose (Standing Forward Bend with the hands on the chair top), lift one leg up and stretch the foot back, creating a "T" like shape with the body. The arms reach forward as you stretch the leg in the air back, finding balance. Focus on one point on front of you, on the chair base or on the floor, that is not moving. Hold and breathe for 1 to 5 deep breaths. Switch Sides.

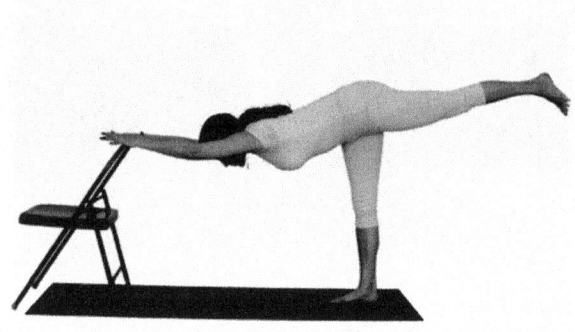

Benefits: Improves leg strength and balance.

Affirmations: I am balanced. I can handle life challenges with inner strength.

Chair Yoga Seated Warrior III,
Virabhadrasana

Sitting tall, lift the arms overhead. Relax the shoulders. Then stretch one leg out and flex the foot. Feel the strength of the legs. See the photos below. You can also stretch one or both arms skywards and hold while the leg is extended (both arms overhead is not shown in photos below). For a gentler adaption, lift one arm and the opposite leg (see the last photo below.)

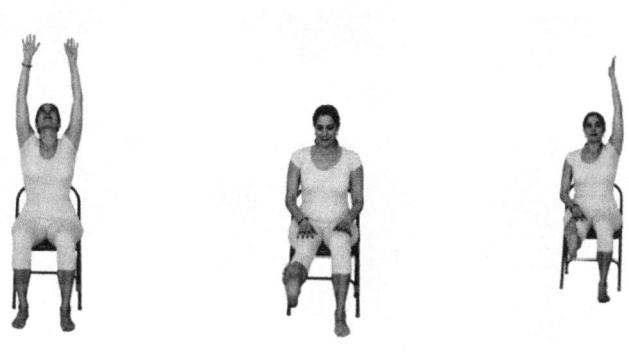

Benefits: Stretches the back and side body. Improves balance, concentration and confidence. The Warrior Poses also are symbols of our inner and outer strength and balance. It can remind you to keep calm and grounded during challenges.

Affirmations: I am strong and focused.

Stork Pose

Stand in Mountain Pose with the feet hip-width apart. Stretch both arms up overhead as you inhale and lift the right foot off the ground, bringing the right knee in line with the right hip joint, or as high as comfortable. Feel the left leg root into the earth. Relax the right upper thigh and shoulders. Hold for 1 to 5 slow, deep breaths. Switch sides. Both arms stretch skywards as you balance and focus the mind.

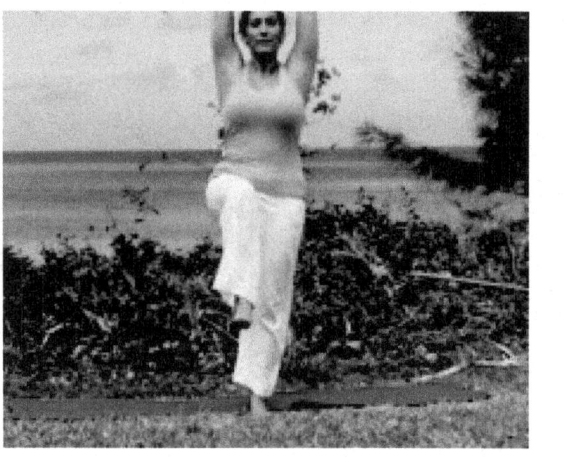

Benefits: Improves balance and concentration and leg strength.

Affirmations: I am balanced. I am focused. I am joyful. I soar to new heights and reach my goals.

Yoga for Everyone!

Chair Yoga Standing Stork Pose

Stand in Mountain Pose to the left side of the chair with the feet hip-width apart. Place the right hand on the top of the chair back for balance support and the left hand on the left hip. Inhale and lift the left foot off the ground, bringing the knee in line with the left hip joint, or as high as comfortable. Feel the standing leg root into the earth. Relax the left upper thigh and shoulders. Hold for 1 to 5 slow, deep breaths.

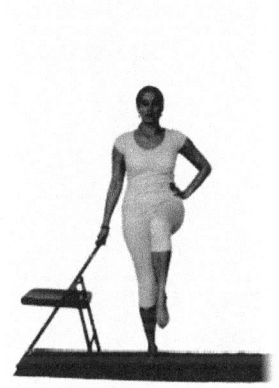

Benefits: Improves balance, stability and concentration. It stretches the spine and waist and brings awareness to the weight shifts on the feet, which can help prevent falls. This pose also strengthens legs.

Affirmation: I am balanced.

Standing Stork Pose Arm Lift Variation

At the same time as you lift the left leg up, or once you find your balance, raise the left arm as well. Hold for 1 to 5 slow, deep breaths. Switch sides. You can also lift both arms overhead and hold as long as you are able.

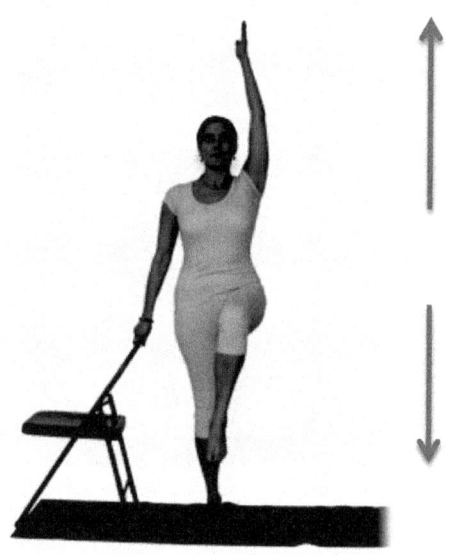

Benefits: Improves balance and concentration. It stretches the spine and waist and brings awareness to the weight shifts on the feet, which can help prevent falls. This pose also strengthens the standing leg.

Chair Yoga Seated Stork Pose

Sit tall in Mountain Pose. Inhale as you stretch the arms skyward. Feel the feet rooting into the earth. Relax the shoulders. Keep the eyes focused on one point that is not moving. Hold for 1 to 5 slow, deep breaths.

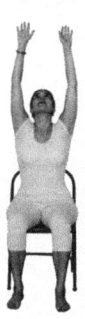

Affirmations: I am filled with *prana* (life energy). I feel alive and well.

"We are not going to change the whole world, but we can change ourselves and feel free as birds. We can be serene even in the midst of calamities and, by our serenity, make others more tranquil. Serenity is contagious. If we smile at someone, he or she will smile back. And a smile costs nothing. We should plague everyone with joy. If we are to die in a minute, why not die happily, laughing?" - Swami Satchidananda, The Yoga Sutras

Half Boat Pose, *Ardha Navasana*

From seated posture, lift the feet and the arms up and balance. Lift out of the core, moving the stomach toward the thighs. Make sure there is no strain in the lower back. Hold on to the back of bent legs, as in the photo below, and try to lift the navel towards the thighs as you balance.

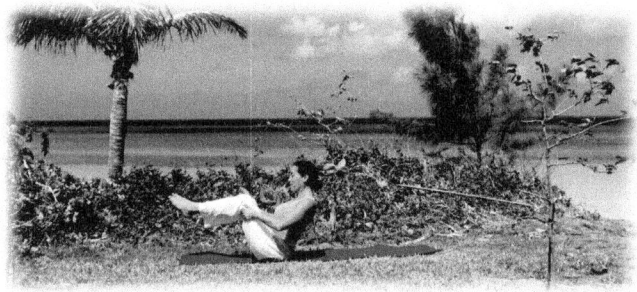

Benefits: Improves core strength and balance.

Full Boat

Start in Half Boat Pose then straighten the legs

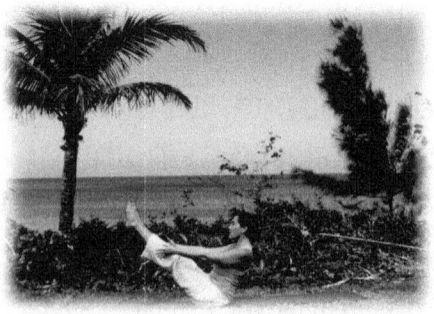

Benefits: Improves core strength and balance.

Chair Yoga Half Boat Pose, *Ardha Navasana*

Hold on to the chair back or base. Sit tall and away from the chair back. Lift the feet and balance on the sits bones. Inhale to lift out of the lower back and lengthen the spine.

If comfortable, lift the feet up in line with the knees. Hold for 1-3 slow, deep breaths. Relax the shoulders and jaw in this pose.

Photo: Chair Yoga Boat Pose with Knees Bent

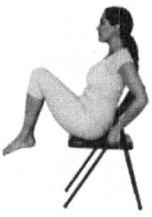

Benefits: Core strength and balance.

Precautions: Do not practice this pose if you have low back pain or a disc injury.

Chair Yoga Half Boat Pose

Photo: Chair Yoga Boat Pose with the Feet In Line With the Knees

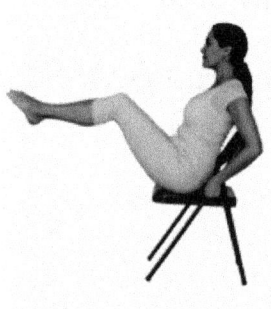

Benefits: Strengthens the core muscles (abdomen) and improves balance both physically and mentally.

Precautions: Do not try this posture if you are pregnant or have lower back injuries or discomfort.

Chair Yoga Boat Pose, *Navasana*

Hold on to the back of the thighs as you lift the spine. Extend the arms out in line with the knees and feet and/or stretch the legs creating a "V" like shape. Hold for 1 to 5 slow, deep breaths. Lift the navel towards the thighs. Relax the shoulders and jaw in this pose.

Photo (left): Hand Behind the Thighs
Photo (right): Arms & Legs Stretched

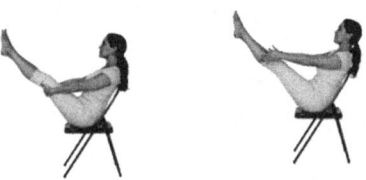

Benefits: Strengthens the core muscles and improves balance both physically and mentally.

Precautions: Do not try this posture if you are pregnant, have lower back pain or disc injuries.

Affirmations: I am balanced. I am strong. I am confident. I live with integrity in my words and actions.

Inversions

Traditional Yoga inversions are postures that turn the body upside down, to allow the legs to be over the heart to benefit the circulatory system, heart, nervous system and lymph system. On the following pages are some Hatha Yoga, Gentle Yoga and Chair Yoga ideas for inversions. You can also rest in Corpse Pose (relaxation pose) instead of inverted the body, which is beneficial as well.

"Calming the mind is yoga. Not just standing on the head."–*Swami Satchidananda*

Shoulderstand, *Sarvangasana*

This posture is a traditional yoga posture practicing after headstand, called "queen of the *asanas*". Lying on your back, lift both legs up and support the back with the hands. Stretch the legs up in the air. The weight is on the elbows and shoulders, not the neck. If able, the legs can be fully vertical with the hips directly over the shoulders (not shown in the photo below), or as much as comfortable. After the Shoulderstand follows the Plough Pose, then Fish Pose (or Bridge Pose, then Fish Pose). Hold steady in the posture, focusing at the throat center for as along as comfortable while you observe the breath. To come out bend the knees, place the hands on the floor and roll out slowly. Then relax in Corpse Pose, *Savasana* and observe.

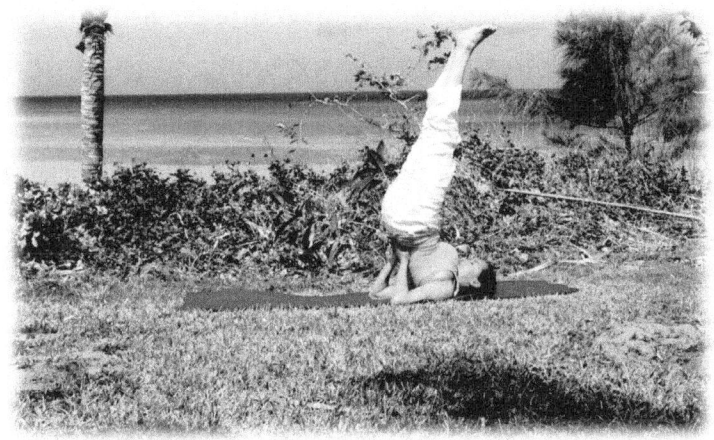

Benefits: Calms the nerves and mind, improves circulation, balances the metabolism and thyroid and improves the immune system.

Precautions: Do not turn the neck in this pose. Do not practice this inversion if you have a detached retina, a neck or shoulder injury, have high blood pressure, are pregnant or on your menstrual cycle.

Half Shoulderstand, *Ardha Sarvangasana*

Lying on your back, lift both legs up and support the back with the hands. Stretch the legs up in the air as the hips lower, keeping the lower back and sacrum area supported by the hands. The weight is on the elbows and shoulders, not the neck. Create an upside down "V" like shape in the body. Hold steady in the posture, focusing at the throat center for as along as comfortable while you observe the breath. To come out bend the knees, place the hands on the floor and roll out slowly. Then relax in Corpse Pose, *Savasana* and observe.

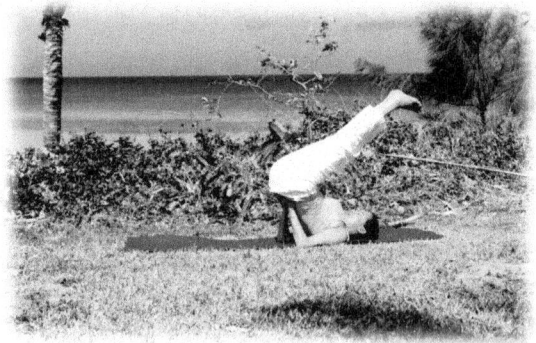

Benefits: Clams the mind, eases varicose veins, and improves circulation, aids digestion, eases fatigue and anxiety. The yogis say this pose increases longevity.

Shoulderstand Precautions: Do not turn your

head in this posture. Do not practice this version of the pose if you are pregnant, on your menstrual cycle, have high blood pressure, back, neck or shoulder injuries or have a detached retina.

Plough Pose, *Halasana*

If Shoulderstand is comfortable, keeping the hands on the back and lower the legs behind the head. If the toes touch the floor, release the hands from the back and interlock the fingers, stretching the arms and hands towards the floor. Do not press the back of the neck into the ground. Make sure there is no weight on the neck and there is no strain.

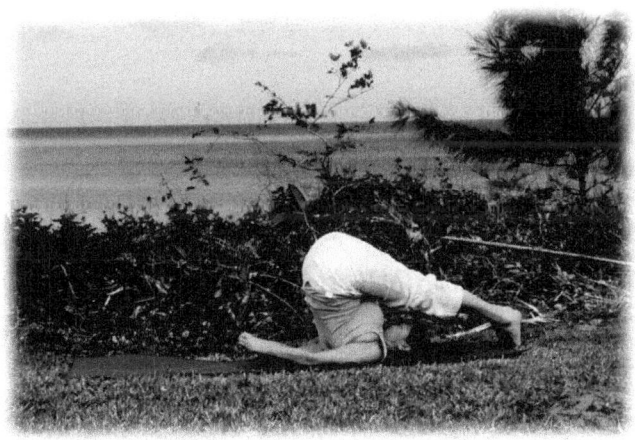

Benefits: Stretches the legs, improves circulation, balances the thyroid gland and metabolism, prevents or eases varicose veins and relaxes the nervous system. This pose rejuvenates the entire body.

Plough Pose Precautions: Do not turn your head in this posture. Do not practice this version of the pose if you are pregnant, have high blood pressure, back, neck or shoulder pain or injuries, or have a detached retina.

Affirmations: I see and enjoy life from different perspectives.

"Begin with little things daily and one day you will be doing things that months back you would have thought impossible."
-Swami Satchidananda

Gentle Yoga Shoulderstand

Legs in the Air Pose

This is a gentle adaption of Shoulderstand, *Sarvangasana*. Lie on your back and stretch the legs up in the air. The arms can relax along side the body. Close the eyes and focus at the center of the throat. Take long, slow deep breaths.

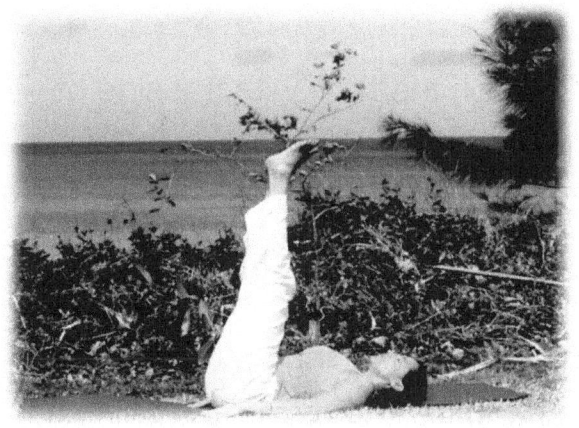

Legs Up the Wall Pose: For more support, support the legs against a wall (not in photo).

Benefits: Assists in circulation, can prevent or ease varicose veins and relaxes the nervous system.

Affirmations: I have plenty of energy.

Legs Up on the Chair Pose

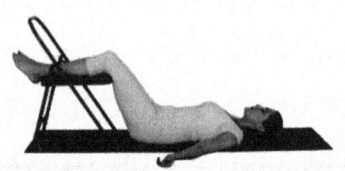

Sit down on the floor with the side of your body facing the chair front. Lower yourself down to your elbows then onto your back, using your hands and arms to support you. Then bring the legs up on the chair. Place the hands about one foot from the hips with the palms facing up towards the sky. Keep the head centered over the spine. Close your eyes. Relax your body and mind. Hold the posture for 3 to 5 minutes or longer if you are comfortable. See the next page for how to come out of the posture safely and gently.

Benefits: Eases lower back pain, can prevent or ease varicose veins, assists circulation, refreshes the body after long flights or stress and relaxes the nervous system.

Precautions: For blood pressure issues and other medical concerns, lie flat on your back (if you

Yoga for Everyone!

are advised to not invert the legs).

Affirmations: I am relaxed and at ease with life. I rest deeply.

How to Come Out of Legs Up on the Chair Pose

To come out of the posture safely and gently from Legs Up on the Chair Pose stretch one or both arms overhead.

Photo below: Stretch one or both arms overhead. Roll to one side (see the photo on the next page). Rest the head on the outstretched arm and pause.

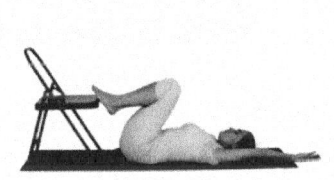

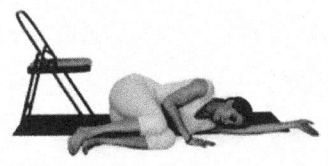

Photos below and on the following page: Use your arms/hands to sit up and the legs to stand. Use the chair base for support.

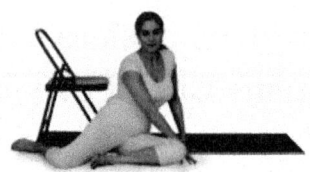

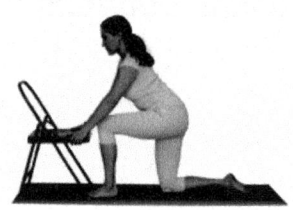

Benefits: Eases lower back pain, assists in circulation and draining lymph from the lower legs and feet towards the heart, relaxes the mind and refreshes the body.

Precautions: Check with your doctor for any medical concerns. If it is difficult or causes strain to lie on the floor, you can rest the feet up on a second chair and rest there. (See the next pose.)

Legs Up on the Chair Pose Upright

Bring the legs up on a second chair in front of you. Lift the arms up overhead and hold 3-6 slow, deep breaths. This is the more active version.

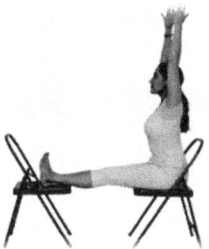

For a more restful version, place the hands on the thighs to rest, as in the photo below.

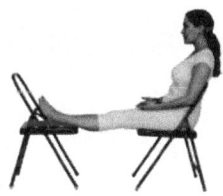

Resting Variation: If the hands are resting on the thighs, the palms can face up towards the sky or faced down if that is more comfortable. Keep the head centered over the spine. You can also place a pillow behind the lower back for support. Close the eyes. Relax your body and mind. Hold for 3 to 10 minutes.

Benefits: The inversions with chairs can have a similar benefit as full yoga inversions (turning the body upside down). It reverses the flow of blood and fluids from standing upright and stimulates the parasympathetic nervous system for calming the nervous system and calming the mind. This also helps reduce jet lag, insomnia and general feelings of stress and exhaustion (mental or physical).

Affirmations: I relax. I am at peace. I have enough energy to d all that I want to in life.

Backbends

Backbends help to ease back tension, relieves dullness, opens the respiratory system to allow for deep breaths, uplifts the mood and brings joy. Restorative Yoga involves the use of props such as blankets, blocks, chairs or pillows so that the body is held in postures with support. This allows for deep relaxation in the body, mind and nervous system and often allows for a longer holding of the posture, since the muscles are relaxed. This is very useful when dealing with fatigue, stress or in need of deep healing and renewal.

The postures in this section show the first Hatha Yoga pose, followed by the Gentle Yoga version of the pose, as well as Chair Yoga supported adaption. Try the version that is most comfortable. This can change from day to day.

"It's very simple. Keep your body as clean as possible, your mind as clear as possible. That's all you need. And do it in anyway you can, in your own way. It doesn't matter. That's why I say 'peaceful body, peaceful mind'. And then you'll be useful. You don't have to become a useful person. You will be useful." –
Swami Satchidananda

Fish Pose, *Matsyasana*

Lie on your back. Place the hands under the thighs, with the palms facing down, as in the photo below. Press the elbows into the floor and if comfortable, lift the heart area and head, to place the top of the head on the floor. The head is upside down. Keep most of the weight in the hands. This posture is traditionally practiced after the Shoulderstand.

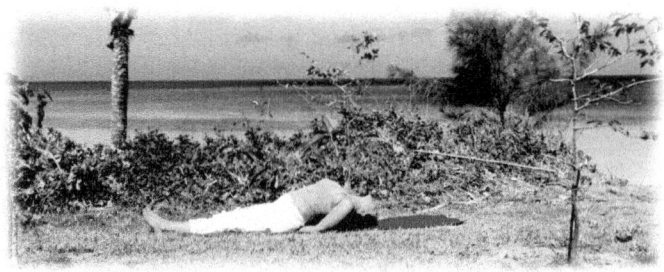

Benefits: Opens the respiratory system to allow for deeper breathing, improves flexibility in the upper back, stretches the entire front of the body, throat and intercostals, relieves dullness and depression, releases back tension and improves the mood. This pose can bring a feeling of joy as the heart area opens.

Precautions: Do not practice this if you have a neck injury. Instead try the Supported Fish.

Affirmations: I open my heart. I flow with life.

Standing Fish Pose, *Matsyasana*

Standing with the feet hip width apart, place the hands on the hips. Inhale as you lift the heart area. Exhale and bring the elbows towards each other without pushing the hips forward. Keep the navel area in towards the spine to stabilize the core. Hold for 2-5 slow, deep breaths. This is a useful adaption for prenatal yoga or for those with an injuries or pre/post surgery and not able to practice lying on the stomach. It is also useful to do at work, as a quick break from the effects of being on the computer for a long period of time.

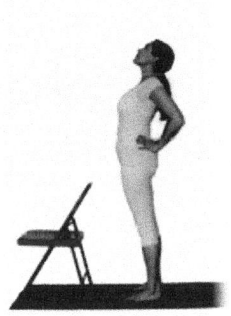

Affirmations: I am safe and supported. I open my heart to love.

Supported Lying Down Fish Pose

Place a rolled towel or blanket on your yoga mat (see photo). Lie down and place the shoulder blades on the blanket. Allow the tops of the shoulders to roll back and down, creating a gentle backbend. This is a restorative version of the Fish Pose. Take 3-8 slow, deep breaths.

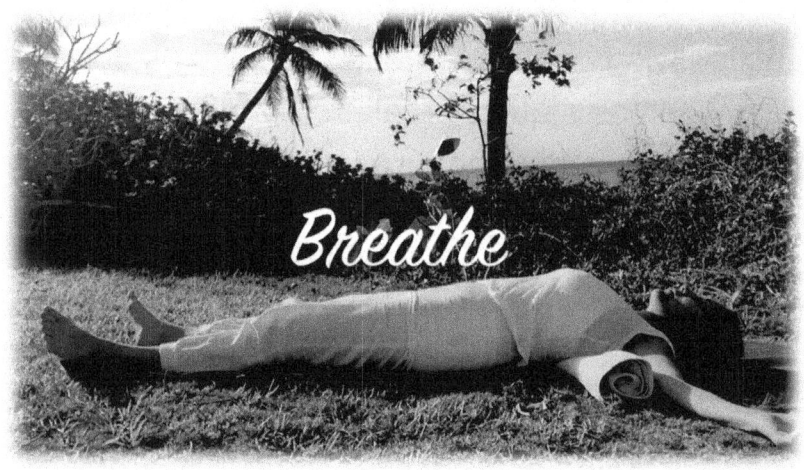

Benefits: Opens the upper back, relaxes the back, neck and shoulders. Fish pose also helps the respiratory system. This pose can bring a feeling of joy and lightheartedness.

Affirmations: I am safe to feel my emotions. I open my heart to love. I am grateful for this life.

Yoga for Everyone!

Seated Chair Yoga Fish Pose,
Matsyasana

(1) Sitting tall, place the hands on the chair base. Lift the sternum and heart area. (2) If able, from there, place the hands on the lower back, with the palms facing the back, or interlock the fingers behind the back as you stretch the hands towards the floor. Feel the heart area lifting, as you take 1-5 slow, deep breaths.

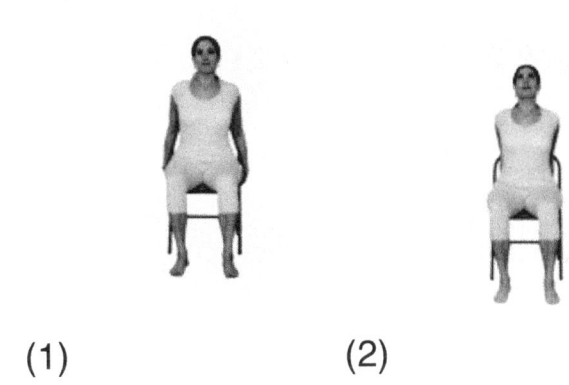

(1)   (2)

Benefits: Opens the respiratory system to allow for deeper breath, improves flexibility in the upper back, relieves dullness, releases back tension and improves the mood.

Chair Yoga Restorative Fish Pose,

Place a rolled yoga mat or towel behind the spine to support the back. Rest the back against the support and stretch the arms to the side. Feel the heart area opening. Take slow, deep breaths. Relax and enjoy this posture.

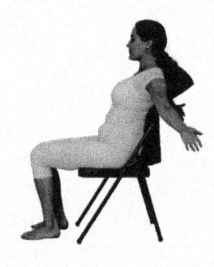

Benefits: Opens the respiratory system to allow for deeper breath, improves flexibility in the upper back, relieves dullness, releases back tension and improves the mood.

Affirmations: I am safe and supported. I trust my inner knowing and listen to my heart. I flow with ease, like a fish in water.

Yoga for Everyone!

Lying down Backbends

Bridge Pose, *Setu Bhandhasana*

Lie on your back with the feet hip-width apart. Place the heels under the knees and point the toes forward. Place the hands along side the hips. As you inhale, press the feet down and lift the hips to create a backbend. The middle back of the head is on the floor (not the back of the neck). In this gentle adaption, as shown in the photo below, the hands hold the sides of the yoga mat, and pull the mat apart, to help lift the heart area and go higher on the shoulders. In the **Hatha Yoga posture**, the fingers interlock under the body and the hands stretch towards the feet. A **Restorative Yoga adaption** is the same posture with a yoga block supporting the sacrum, with the arms relaxed.

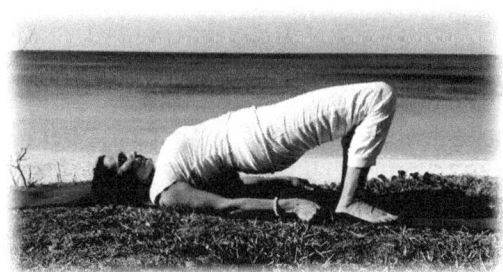

Benefits: Strengthens the back, hamstrings and buttocks, increases flexibility in the back, stretches the abdomen and removes dullness.

Supported Cobra Pose/"Sphinx Pose", *Salamba Bhujanasana*

Lying down on the stomach, place the elbows under the shoulders and the hands in line with the elbows. Lift the heart area on the inhalation and hold the pose for 1-5 slow, deep breaths. Feel as if you are pulling the floor towards you with the forearms and relax the shoulders.

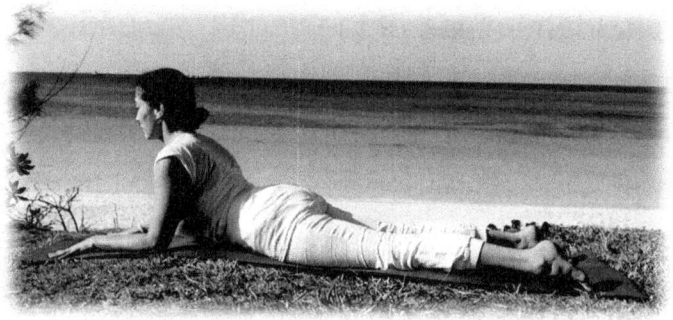

Benefits: Strengthens the lower back and arms, increases flexibility, massages the abdomen, improves menstrual symptoms and elevates the mood. Backbends are heart openers and can bring joy or release stuck emotions in the heart center.

Precautions: Gently move the tailbone towards the earth (a slight tilt of the pelvis forward, moving the lower navel in towards the spine), so that you do not over arch the back and stabilize the core.

Affirmations: I am stable and strong.

Cobra Pose, *Bhujangasana*

Lying down on the stomach, place the hands under the shoulders. Inhale as you lift the heart and chest off the floor. Hold for 1-5 slow, deep breaths.

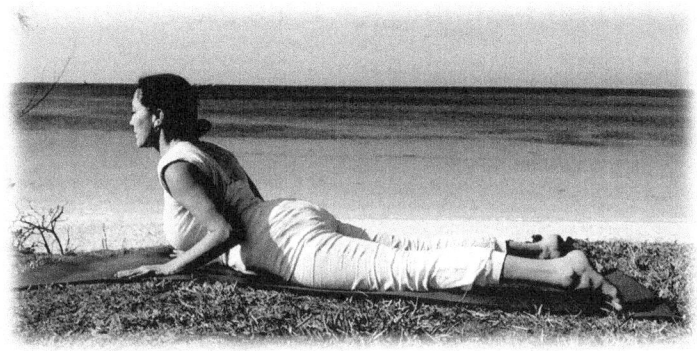

Benefits: Strengthens the lower back and increases flexibility in the the upper back, massages the digestive organs and stomach, improves the mood and reduces menstrual symptoms.

Precautions: Do not practice the backbends lying on the stomach if you are pregnant.

Affirmations: I am flexible and strong. I move with grace and ease.

Chair Yoga Cobra Pose

See Chair Yoga Fish Pose on the previous pages.

Half Locust Pose, *Ardha Salabhasana*

Lying face down with the forehead resting on the hands, lift one leg as you lengthen the toes back. Hold and breathe for 1-4 slow, deep breaths. Switch sides.

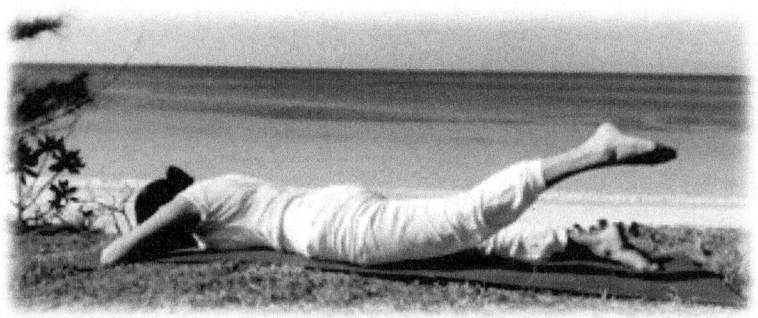

Benefits: Strengthens the entire back, legs and buttocks, and can ease digestion.

Precautions: Do not practice if pregnant (see the Standing Locust Pose in the following pages for prenatal variations).

Affirmations: I am strong. I am supported.

Full Locust Pose, *Salabhasana*

Lying face down with the forehead resting on the hands, take a few slow breaths and relax. Then bring your arms along side your legs. Lift the chest, arms and legs up. Hold and enjoy for 1-4 slow, deep breaths as you stretch the arms, fingers, legs and toes back.

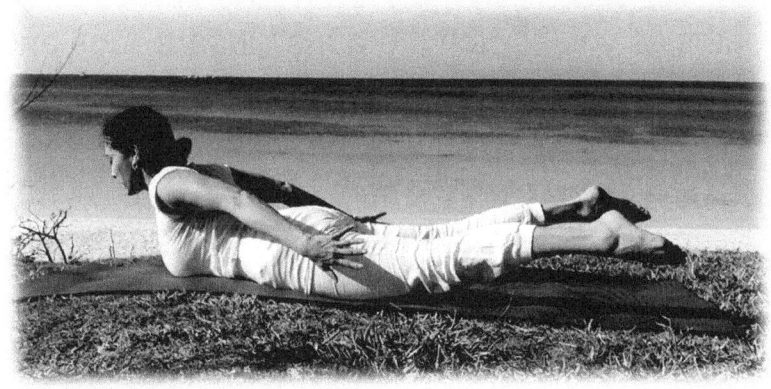

Benefits: Strengthens the entire back, legs and buttocks, and can ease digestion.

Precautions: Do not practice if pregnant (see below for prenatal variations).

Affirmations: I am strong in both body and mind. I soar to new heights with every breath.

Full Locust Pose Variation,
Salabhasana

Lying face down with the forehead resting on the hands, take a few slow breaths and relax. Then interlock the fingers behind your back. Lift the chest, arms and legs up as you stretch the hands back. Hold and enjoy 1-4 slow, deep breaths as you stretch the arms, fingers, legs and toes back.

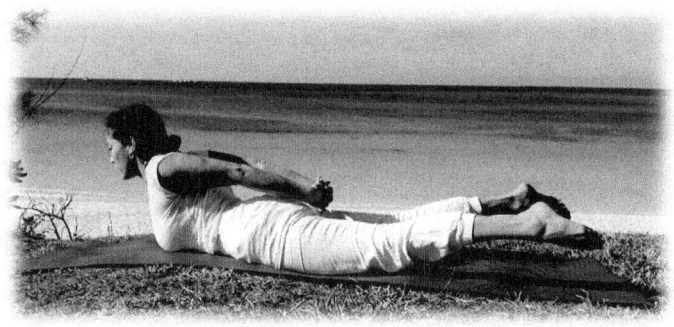

Benefits: Strengthens the entire back, legs and buttocks, and can ease digestion. This variation opens the shoulder area and relieves shoulder and upper back tension.

Precautions: Do not practice if pregnant (see below for prenatal variations).

Affirmations: I am strong in both body and mind. I soar to new heights with every breath.

Standing Chair Yoga Locust Pose, *Salabhasana*

Stand behind the chair with the feet hip-width apart. Balance the weight equally on both feet. Move your tailbone towards the floor as you move the navel area in towards the spine. Lift the spine as you extend one leg/foot back. Keep your toes on the floor, if needed, and your hands on the chair, or release one hand from the chair, and lift the arm overhead (see the following page). Hold for 3 to 5 slow, deep breaths while stretching the back leg. Switch sides.

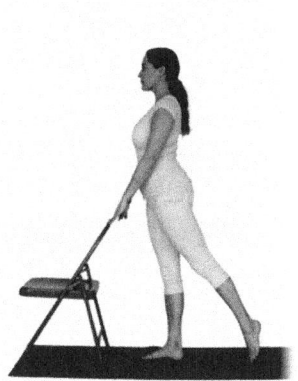

Benefits: Strengthens the legs and buttocks, increases the range of motion in the hips.

Affirmations: I am balanced. I am strong.

Balancing Standing Chair Yoga
Locust Pose, *Ardha Salabhasana*

While in Locust Pose, inhale as you lift one or both arms up. Exhale as you lower. Repeat 2x. Or hold and balance with both arms overhead. Enjoy 3 to 5 slow, deep breaths as you hold the posture. Keep the shoulders relaxed and the area below the navel moving slightly in towards the spine so that the pelvis is in a neutral position

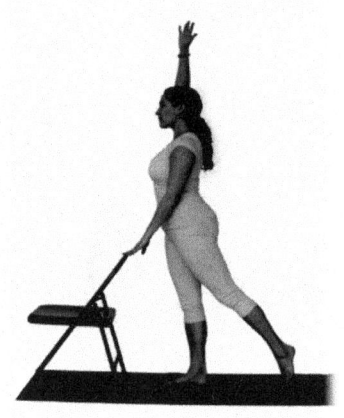

Locust With One Arm Up

Benefits: Strengthens the legs and buttocks, increases the range of motion in the hips. This can be a prenatal modification for the Locust Pose

Bow Pose, *Dhanurasana*

Lying on your stomach, bend the knees and hold the ankles (or feet). Keep the thighs rotating in towards each other and the tailbone gently moving towards the earth (so that you keep the low back stable). Press the hands into the ankles or feet as you press the feet or ankles back into the hands, while you lift your chest and thighs off the floor. Hold for 1-5 slow, deep breaths.

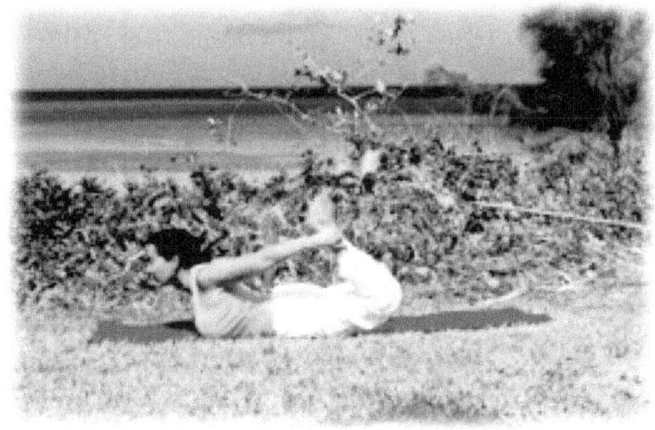

Benefits: Opens the upper back, stretches the entire front of the body, ankles, chest and quadriceps, improves posture and strengthens the back muscles. Backbends such as this one also improve your mood and bring joy, easing feelings of dullness and depression.

<u>**Affirmations:**</u> I open my heart to life.

Standing Variation of Half Bow Pose,

Cosmic Dancer, *Natarajasana*

If getting up and down on the floor, or lying on the stomach is not comfortable, you can try this version of the backbend. Standing in Mountain Pose, (place one hand on a chair top if you need), bend the right knee and hold the right foot behind you with the left hand. If the hand does not touch the foot comfortably, place the right hand on the hip, keeping the back knee bent. Inhale as you lift the chest bone (sternum) up. Keep the navel in towards the spine, to stabilize the low back. Hold and balance for 1-5 slow, deep breaths. The photo below and the following page shows different variations of the pose.

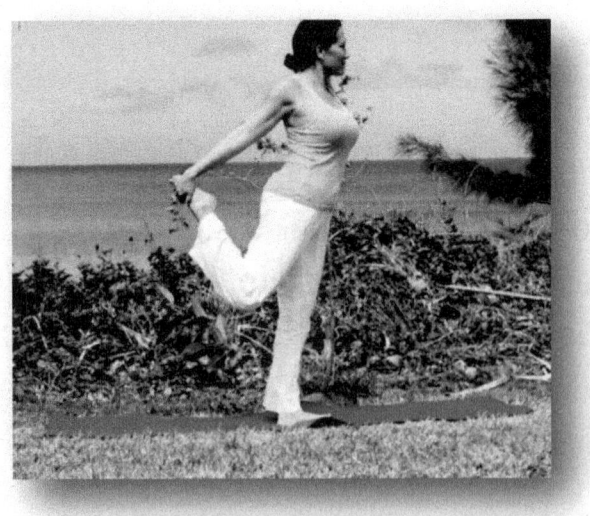

Yoga for Everyone!

Standing Variation of Half Bow Pose/Cosmic Dancer, *Natarajasana*

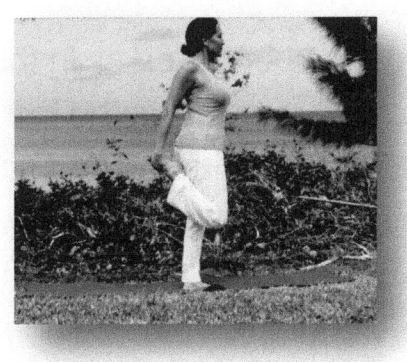

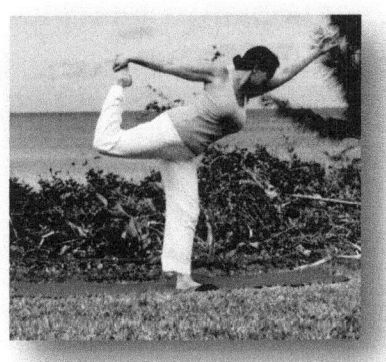

Benefits: Stretches the quadriceps, chest, groins and front of the body, strengthens the legs and improves balance and the ability to focus the mind.

Affirmations: I am balanced. I feel vital.

Seated Chair Yoga Half Bow Pose,
Ardha Dhanurasana

If the chair has open sides as in the photo below, turn the body to the side so that both legs and feet are on one the side of the chair, with the side body (waist) facing the chair back. Hold onto the outside foot with the outside hand (the hand and foot furthest away from the chair back). Hold onto your pants or use a yoga belt if needed. You can also lift the foot up and place the hand on the hip if holding the foot or belt is not accessible. Switch sides and hold as long as comfortable.

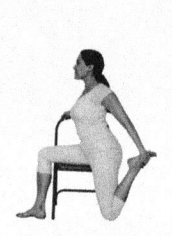

Benefits: Opens the upper back and stretches the quadriceps and front of the thigh. Backbends such as this one also improve your mood and bring joy, easing feelings of dullness.

Affirmation: I open my heart to life.

Lying Down Bound Angle Pose
Backbend, *Supta Baddha Konasana*

Lying on your back, bend the knees and bring the bottoms of the feet together. Inhale deeply. As you exhale release the knees away from each other, towards the earth, releasing the legs into a diamond shape. Support the outer knees if you need with blankets, folded towels or yoga blocks. As in this photo, you can place a rolled towel (or second yoga mat rolled up) horizontal, under the shoulder blades to add a restorative backbend.

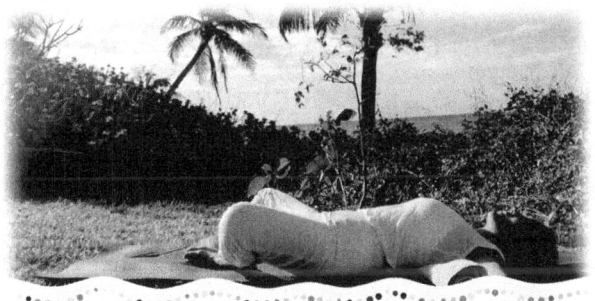

Supta Baddha Konasana (Bound Angle Pose)

Benefits: Stretches the spine and improves flexibility in the inner thighs, groins and the knees. The rolled blanket under the upper back helps ease back tension, opens the upper back and allows for a more easeful breath. This pose can ease menstrual discomfort.

Spinal Twists

Spinal twists are calming for the nerves and the mind. Twists also aid digestion, ease tension and increase flexibility.

Seated Spinal Twist,
Ardha Matsyendrasana

Sitting tall, stretch the legs out. Place your right foot over the left shin or knee area, keeping the weight even between the sits bones. Bend the left leg and place the foot by the right buttocks. Inhale as you sit tall. Exhale as your twist to the right and place your right hand behind the back. Bring the left hand to the right outer thigh or hug the outer thigh, as comfortable. Hold for 1-5 slow, deep breaths. Switch sides.

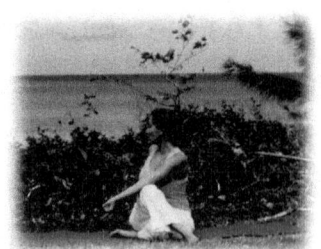

Benefits: Releases back tension, helps the digestive organs and calms the nervous system. Increases spinal flexibility.

Precautions: If pregnant, for all twists, do not twist through the torso (belly). Twist only from the area above the ribcage (all trimesters). For neck pain, keep the head facing forward, or as is comfortable.

Gentle Seated Half Spinal Twist, *Ardha Matsyendrasana*

Sitting tall, stretch the legs out. Place your right foot over the left shin or knee area, keeping the weight even between the sits bones. Inhale as you sit tall. Exhale as your twist to the right and place your right hand behind the back. Bring your left hand outside the right outer thigh or hug the outer thigh, as comfortable. Hold for 1-5 slow, deep breaths. Switch sides.

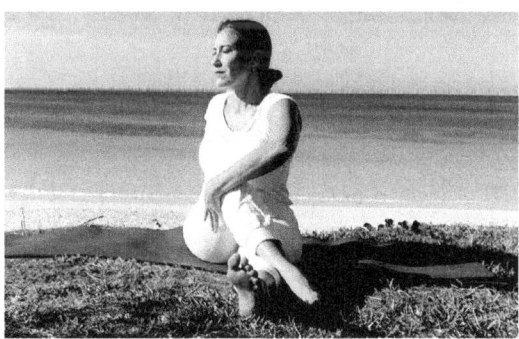

Benefits: Relaxes, lengthens and realigns the spine, massages the abdominal organs.

Lying Down Spinal Twist

Lying on your back, place the arms in a "T" like shape, with the hands in line with the shoulders. Bend the knees bring the knees into the chest. Inhale deeply. As you exhale, release both knees to the right as you roll the head to the left. Hold for 1-5 slow, deep breaths. Switch sides.

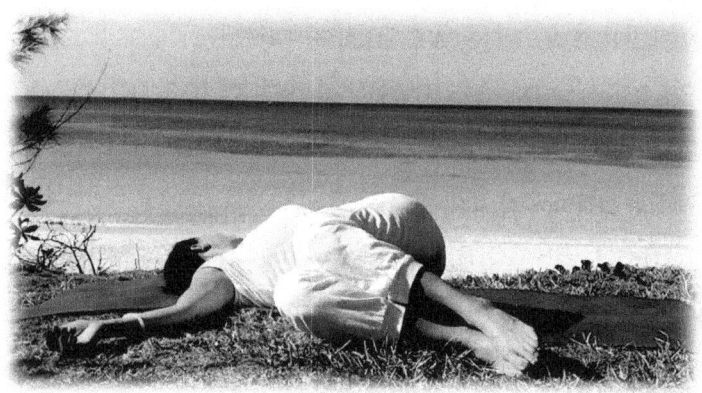

Benefits: Releases back tension, helps the digestive organs and calms the nervous system. Increases spinal flexibility

Affirmations: I digest my food and emotions in a healthy way. I move with ease. My body supports me and is flexible and strong. I am grateful to breathe. I relax with every breath.

Lying Down Gentle Spinal Twist

Lying on your back, place the arms in a "T" like shape, with the hands in line with the shoulders. Bend the knees and place the feet together on the floor. Inhale deeply. As you exhale, release both knees to the left as you roll the head to the right. Hold for 1-5 slow, deep breaths. Switch sides.

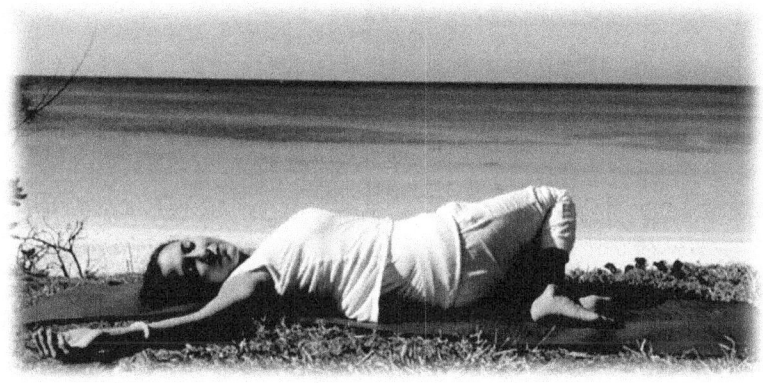

Benefits: Releases back tension, helps the digestive organs and calms the nervous system. Increases spinal flexibility

Affirmations: I digest my food and emotions in a healthy way. I move with ease. My body supports me and is flexible and strong. I am grateful to breathe. I relax with every breath.

Hugging Twist

Sitting in a cross-legged seat or in a chair, cross the left arm over the right and give yourself a big hug. Gently rock the upper body side to side several times. Switch sides. Place the right arm over the left and repeat.

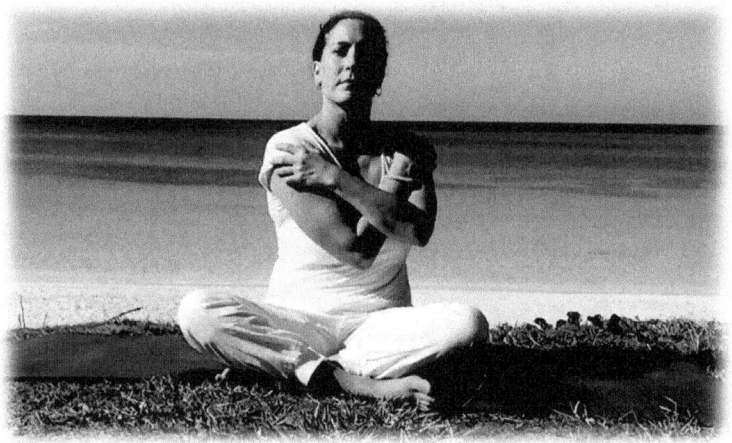

Benefits: Releases upper back tension and relaxes the shoulders.

Affirmations: I love and respect myself. I nurture myself and take care of my body.

Lying Down Rocking Twist

Lie down on your back and hugs the knees to the chest. Gently rock the body side to side several times. Allow the head to roll opposite way of the legs.

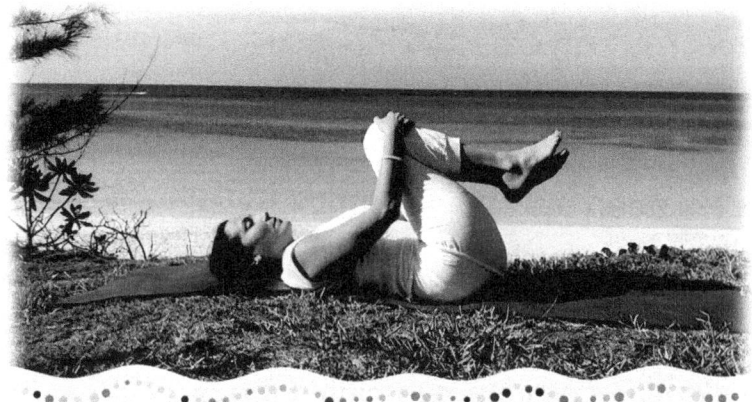

Rocking Twist: massage the back

Benefits: Releases back tension and is calming.

Chair Yoga Spinal Twist, *Ardha Matsyendrasana*

Inhale as you sit tall. Exhale as you twist to one side. Keep the head centered over the spine and twist gently and evenly throughout the entire spine. You can cross your legs fully or just the ankles. See the next page for photos showing details about how to get into the posture. Inhale as you lengthen the spine (sit tall). Exhale as you gently twist. Hold for 1 to 5 deep breaths.

Benefits: Releases back tension, massages the digestive organs and calms the nervous system. Increases spinal flexibility, lengthens, realigns and relaxes the spine.

Precautions: If pregnant, for all twists, do not twist through the torso (belly). Twist only from the area above the ribcage (all trimesters). For whiplash or neck pain, keep the head facing forward or as comfortable.

Affirmations: I digest my food and emotions in a healthy way. I move with ease. My body supports me and is flexible and strong. I am grateful to breathe and relax with every breath.

Getting into the Chair Yoga
Seated Spinal Twist

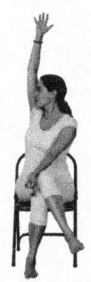

Inhale as you lift the right arm.
Exhale as you twist to the right.

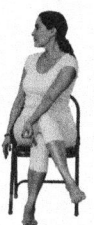   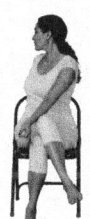

Arm by the Chair Side   Arm by the Chair Back

Flow Like a River: Hatha Yoga Inspiration from the Ganges

I traveled through Northern India in 2016 with my father. When I reached the Ganges River in Rishikesh, home to many yoga ashrams, I was captivated by the quality of the river currents as I sat and watched the river flow downstream.

The river flowed continuously—some days more rough than others—yet there was always a calmness, gracefulness and gentle flow to it as the currents passed me by. Solid earthen hills towered behind the "Mother Ganges," as the river is endearingly called, creating a perfect balance of the elements: water, earth, fire (the sun rising behind the river) and air (the gentle breeze).

I was reminded that this is the exact quality of grace, ease and balance we can create in our own bodies, minds and lives with the practice of Hatha Yoga. In Sanskrit, Hatha Yoga translates to sun *(ha)* and moon *(tha)* union, creating balance of opposites.

While in Rishikesh, I practiced yoga daily before sunrise, as the yogis do, to maximize the energy and alignment of the sun and to achieve the calmness of the mind in the auspicious hours *(amrit vela)*. At the Sivananda Yoga Divine Life Society ashram where I was staying, I would practice on the porch where the great yogi Swami Sivananda lived and practiced himself.

Each day, I would practice the ancient techniques of *pranayama* (breathing practices) for balance and energy and to prepare the mind for concentration *(dharana)*. Afterwards, I would sit in stillness, observing the breath, heading towards a meditative state *(dhyana)* for inner peace, clarity and perhaps even a taste of bliss.

Then, after meditation, just as the sun was rising behind the Ganges (at the early 5:20 a.m. hour) I would start my Sun Salutations *Surya Namaskar)* to warm the body up for the main yoga postures, which provide radiant health, vitality, strength and flexibility in the body and mind.

As a yoga instructor teaching daily to companies in the Bay Area, California, I was inspired to share the sequence I was practicing with my students and others, so that more people can feel their own energy flow like a river— afterwards allowing their mind to be still and calm.

"Be still like a mountain and flow like a great river." ~ Lao Tzu

"Flow Like a River"
Hatha Yoga Sequence on the Ganges

Modify all postures so that your body is comfortable, and make sure that there is no strain or pain. Take breaks when you need (rest on your back in corpse pose, called *savasana*). For those needing to adapt this sequence in a chair or wheelchair, you can learn more ideas in my book, SunLight Chair Yoga: yoga for everyone! or in the previous sections of this book.

Warm Ups, heating like the sun

Warm up with Sun Salutations (*Surya Namaskar*), a series of 12 postures in sync and flowing with your breath. Try it facing the sun, outside. (See the Sun Salutations in this book.)

Standing Flow Sequence, moving like a river

These standing postures increase leg strength, opens the hips, bring stability and balance to the body and mind and stretches the back. You can flow from one posture to the next, or take breaks in between by pausing in Mountain Pose

Yoga for Everyone!

(Tadasana), standing with your feet together and balancing the weight on both feet.

Warrior Posture, *Virabhadrasna*

Place your feet three to four feet apart. Bend your front leg and keep the back leg straight, pressing the back heel and foot evenly into the earth. Turn the hips and torso to face the front leg. Stretch the arms up overhead and if able, place the palms together, while you keep the face and shoulders relaxed.

Focus the eyes in front of you on one point or gazing skywards, towards the hands.

Hold for three to five slow, deep breaths.

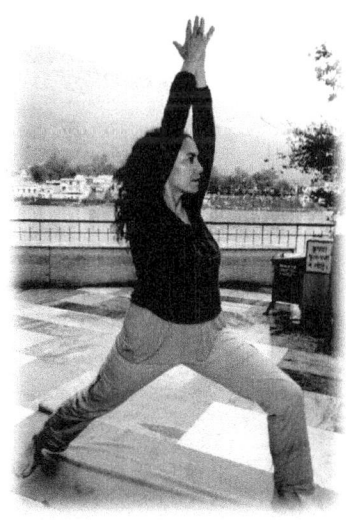

Feel your strength, focus and determination as a peaceful warrior, as you ground your feet into the earth while lifting your heart up to the heavens.

Warrior Pose Alignment tips:

~ Make sure that the front knee does not go past your front heel.

~ Evenly press the inner and outer heels of your back foot into the ground.

Modify the shoulders and arms by keeping the hands shoulder width apart overhead as needed, or bring the hands out in front of you instead of overhead.

Benefits: Increases leg strength, balance, supports the knee joints, and mentally brings joy, positivity, focus, determination and confidence.

Affirmations: I am flexible. My life flows with ease. I am energized.

Warrior Pose: Hip and Shoulder Opening Variation

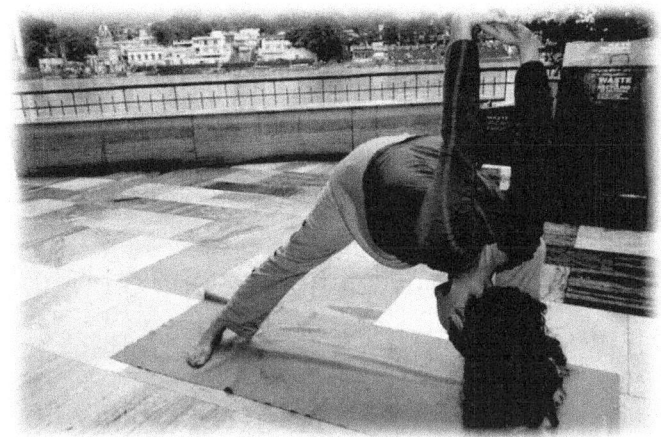

From Warrior Pose, interlock the fingers behind you. Inhale as you lift the heart up towards the sky and simultaneously stretch the hands towards the earth (this opens the chest, upper back and shoulders). As you exhale, bend at the hips and relax the top of the head toward the inside (big toe side) of the front foot.

Keep pressing the back foot evenly into the earth as in Warrior Pose. Hold for three to five slow, deep breaths. To come out of the posture, ground the back foot (press it into the earth), inhale as you rise back up to Warrior Pose. Repeat on the second side or continue with the next few poses as a flow sequence by keeping the same foot forward for all postures.

Repeat the whole sequence on the other side.

Yoga practice, just like life, is full of options. You can also flow back and forth between the two postures in the photos above. For example, inhale to Warrior Pose, and then exhale in to the hip and shoulder opening variation.

Repeat three to five times, keeping both feet rooting into the earth.

Intense Side Stretch Pose,
Parsvottanasana

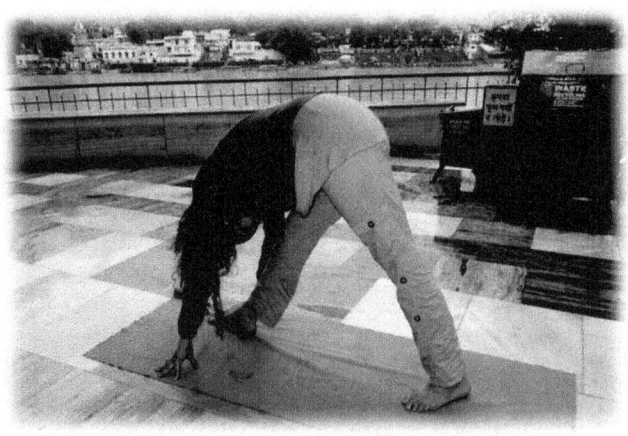

Place your feet three to four feet apart. Straighten your front leg. Inhale as you stretch the arms up towards the sky. Exhale and stretch the spine away from the hips and towards the front leg. Then release the hands to the front leg or floor along side the legs or feet (you can also use two yoga blocks to support the hands or place the hands on a chair or table out in front of you). Hold and breath for three to five slow, deep, rhythmic breaths. Relax into the pose.

Modify the posture by bending the front leg slightly, as needed so that there is no strain.

Benefits: This posture stretches the legs, hamstrings and spine (good for runners and athletes).

Extended Side Angle Pose from Warrior

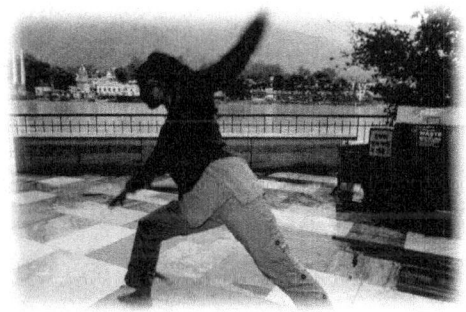

From Warrior Pose open the hips to face forward (no longer towards the front thigh). Stretch the arms in, away from the heart (in a T shape). You can hold there (Warrior II Pose) for three to five slow, deep breaths. As you exhale stretch the spine over your front (bent knee) leg, while keeping the chest facing forward.

Release the front hand to rest on the front thigh or floor (in front or behind the front leg). Hold for three to five slow, relaxed breaths. Keep the weight even on both feet. To come out of the posture, press your back foot into the earth and inhale to rise up back to Warrior II (you can also repeat the sequence again if you want a more vigorous practice).

Reverse Warrior Pose

From Extended Side Angle, go back into Warrior II Pose (arms stretch out in a T shape). Place your back hand on the back thigh (or outer shin) as you exhale, while you stretch the top arm over the top ear, creating a crescent moon shape or gentle curve with your spine. Keep the weight even in both feet as in Warrior I and hold for three to five slow deep breaths. Inhale to come out the posture. See the photo below.

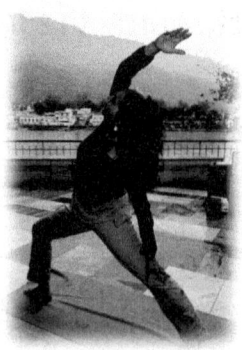

Yoga for Everyone!

Rest in Mountain Pose *(Tadasana)* with your feet together as you evenly distribute the weight between both feet. Pause and feel the effects of the standing postures.

Seated Postures, rooting like a mountain

Wide Leg Seated Forward Bend, *Uppavistha Konasana*

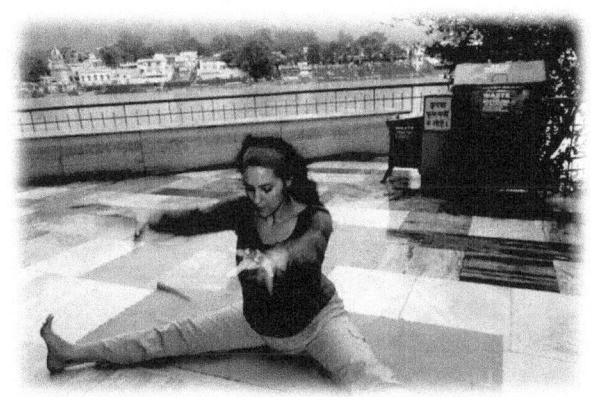

Stretch your legs apart, as wide as comfortable, without causing strain. Press the top back of each thigh evenly into the earth. Sit on a cushion or folded towel as needed to support the back. Inhale as you stretch the arms overhead. Exhale and fold forward placing your hands on the floor, thighs, holding the big toes or using yoga blocks in front of you (for more support).

Alignment tips:

~ Do not let the buttocks or thighs lift off the floor as you fold forward.

~ Keep the middle of the knees and the toes facing skywards.

Seated Side Bending from Wide Angle Pose

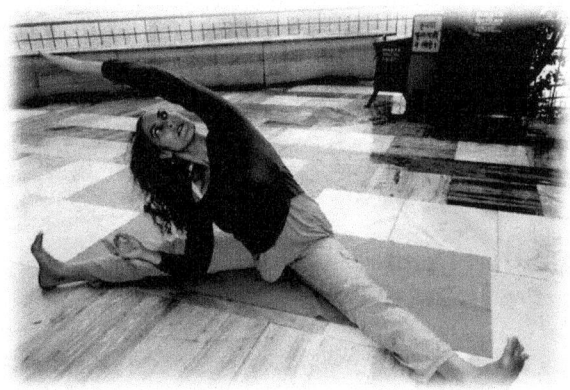

Stretch your legs apart, as wide as comfortable, without causing strain. Press the top back of each thigh evenly into the earth. Sit on a cushion or folded towel as needed to support the back. Inhale as you stretch the arms overhead. Exhale and gently curve the spine to one side, placing the bottom arm in front of the thigh (or resting it on a yoga block for more support). As a modification you can also place the bottom hand on the floor.

Gently turn the spine and chest towards the sky, allow the neck to follow and look towards the top arm. (If there is any strain in the neck, look forward or down instead.) Hold for three to five slow breaths. Switch sides.

Seated Side Bending in Wide Angle Pose Alignment tips:

~ Only bend sideways as far as comfortable, while keeping both thighs and buttocks evenly pressing into the earth.

~ Have all the toes facing skywards (do not let the legs roll outwards).

Benefits: Stretches the legs, side body and opens the side ribs to give a feeling of expansion and more room to breath easily and freely. This lateral bend increases flexibility of the spine and legs.

Wide Leg Seated Spinal Twist

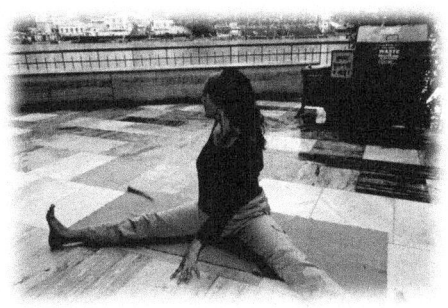

Stretch your legs apart, as wide as comfortable, without causing strain. Press the top back of each thigh evenly into the earth. Sit on a cushion or folded towel as needed to support the back. Inhale as you stretch the arms overhead. Exhale and gently twist to one side while keeping the spine lengthening skywards. Place one hand behind you and one hand in front of you as in the photo below. Inhale as you sit tall, and exhale as you twist. Repeat for three to five slow, deep breaths and then switch sides.

Benefits: Helps the digestive organs, eases back tension and calms the nerves.

Standing Balance Pose

Now that you created flexibility, balance, stability and strength in the body and mind you can end with a one-legged balance posture to improve your mental concentration.

Natarajasana in Sanskrit is the cosmic dancer. This is symbolic of the dance of the soul: birth, life, transformation or death (or what the dance of life means to you). In this posture you can find stability and also have some fun in the process. If you fall or don't feel very graceful, that too is a dance, so enjoy it!

Yoga for Everyone!

Benefits: helps improve your concentration and focus. This posture also creates balance in the body and helps bring stability to the joints and is an upper back and shoulder opener (backbend). Symbolically this pose can help your find ease and balance even in the constant movement of life.

Cosmic Dancer Pose *Natarajasana*

Balance on two feet. Shift the weight to one foot. Hold on to one foot or as a modification you can hold onto your pants or use a yoga belt as in the photo below.

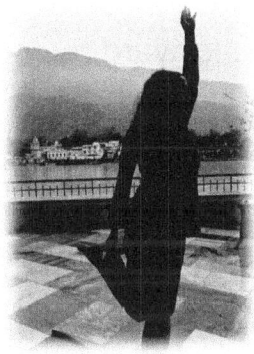

As you hold the foot or pants, lift the back foot up and press it back away from the body. While you do this stretch the other arm overhead, placing the upper arm by the ear, or even moving the arm towards the back of the head. Find your breath and breathe into the opening and expansion of the chest and upper back.

Cosmic Dancer Variation

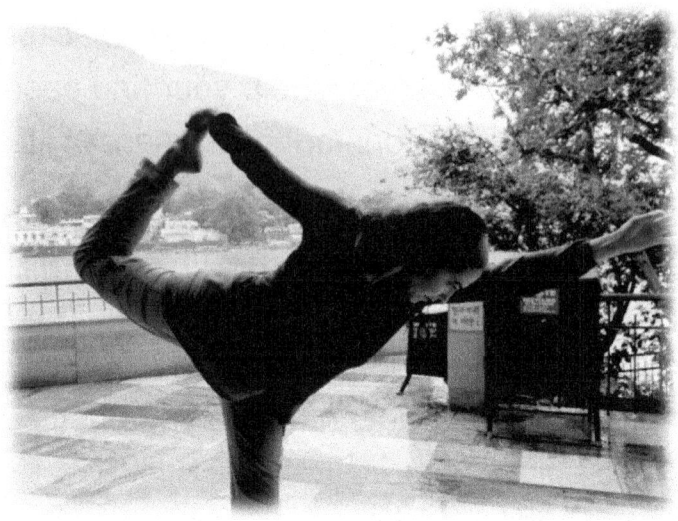

Tilt the pelvis forward trying to keep the back thigh lifting in line with the front arm ahead of you. Do your best to create a parallel line between the back thigh and front arm. Hold for three to five slow deep breaths while keeping the eyes focused on one point in front of you. Inhale and slowly ease out. Switch sides.

Final Relaxation

Lie on your back in Corpse Pose, *Savasana*. Places the feet two to three feet apart, and the arms a few inches from your hips. The palms face skywards. Relax for 10 minutes. Observe each part of the body relax. Then watch the breath and allow all thoughts to flow in and out, just like currents in a river. Be a silent witness to the relaxation process. Let the mind rest deep within. Enjoy the deep stillness and peace beneath and between the waves of the mind.

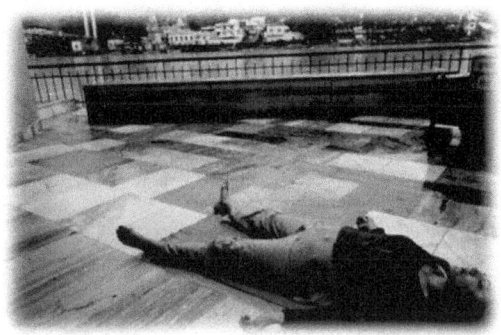

To come out of *Savasana* bring the knees into the chest, roll to the right side and pause. Slowly push off your hands to ease yourself sitting upright in a cross-legged seat. Meditate on the breath for two to 31 minutes. Chant three *"AUMS"* ॐ Focus at the point between the eyebrows.

"Serve, Love, Give, Purify, Meditate, Realize." –Swami Sivananda

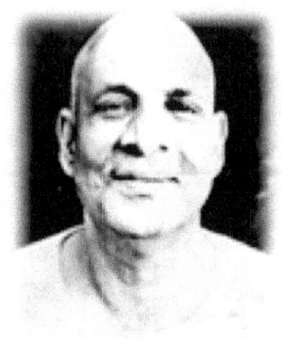

Swami Sivananda

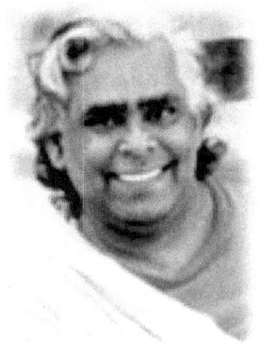

Swami Vishnudevananda

Sivananda Yoga-Chair Yoga

4

In Chapter4, Sivananda Yoga in Chairs

- Sivananda Yoga Sequence
- *Pranayama* (Breathing)
- Sun Salutations
  - Chair Yoga Adaptions
- 12 Yoga *Asanas* (Poses)
  - Chair Yoga Adaptions
- Deep Relaxation
- Sivananda Yoga Sequence, Adapted Using Chairs

Sivananda Yoga Sequence Modified in Chairs

Swami Sivananda was a great yoga master and Guru to many. The teachings of Sivananda are summarized in these six words: Serve, Love, Give, Purify, Meditate, Realize. Swami Vishnudevananda was a disciple of Sivananda and founder of the International Sivananda Yoga Vedanta Centers and Ashrams.

A basic Sivananda class consists of relaxation *(savasana),* breathing exercises (*pranayama)*, Sun Salutations *(Surya Namaskar)*, and 12 main yoga postures *(asanas).* Variations of these postures are usually included, and others may be added. For more extensive reading on this lineage of yoga and to see photos of all of the main postures in this sequence, visit: www.sivanandasf.org

Based on my experience as a certified Sivananda Yoga instructor since 1995, many people need to adapt the traditional postures to make it accessible. This chapter suggests ways to modify yoga *asanas* in the Sivananda Yoga sequence, for those needing to use chairs and in wheelchairs, as support during the practice. For yoga instructors, this chapter can give you ideas how to offer Chair Yoga adaptions for one student in a group class (if they are not able to sit or lie down on the floor for certain postures), or to offer this sequence in class for all of the students (for Chair Yoga classes).

The need for Chair Yoga adaptions can be due to injury, illness, disability, pre or post surgery, limited mobility, prenatal yoga adaptions or other reasons. Any chair you have may have to suffice, so you may need to be creative. If the chair you have isn't stable you can put the chair against the wall.

Sivananda Yoga Sequence (without chairs)

- Breathing Exercises *(Pranayama)*
- Sun Salutations, *Surya Namaskar* (3-6x)
- Headstand *(Sirshasana)*
    - o Or Child's Pose and/or Dolphin Pose
- Shoulderstand *(Sarvangasana)*
    - o Or Legs Up the Wall or Chair Pose
- Plough *(Halasana)*
- Fish *(Matsyasana)*
- Forward bend *(Paschimothanasana)*
- Cobra *(Bhujangasana)*

- Locust *(Shalabhasana)*
- Bow *(Dhanurasana)*
- Spinal Twist (*Ardha Matsyendrasana)*
- Crow pose *(Kakasana)* or Tree Pose *(Vrksasana)*
- Standing Forward Bend *(Pada Hasthasana)*
- Triangle *(Trikonasana)*
- *Corpse Pose (Savasana)*
  - ○ Autosuggestion and Deep Relaxation

Sivananda Yoga Sequence in Chairs

This chapter offers suggestions for the Sivannada Yoga sequence adapted in chairs, as taught in my SunLight Chair Yoga Teacher Trainings.

Pranayama

Yogic breathing exercises, called *pranayama* in Sanskrit, can be practiced the same sitting in a chair or wheelchair, instead of cross-legged on the floor as traditionally done. You can also modify the breathing exercises for pregnancy, health conditions or other concerns by not holding the breath (retention) or as needed specific to your students needs. If you are familiar with the full Sivananda Yoga sequence, you can practice the full *pranayama* exercises as taught in class. This chapter with show some modified breathing exercises and postures.

For example, during Alternative Nostril Breath *(Anuloma Viloma)* instead of holding the breath as usually taught, you can instead simple inhale the left nostril, exhale the right nostril, then inhale through the right nostril and exhale through the left as one round, which is without breath retention. If you have arthritis or other conditions that prevent the comfortable use of the right hand in *Vishnu Mudra* (or any *mudra*) you can block the nostrils with the palm flat using the index fingers or as able (see the photos on the following page).

Slow deep breathing, full yogic breath (three part breath) exercise, or simple alternative nostril breath without holding the breath (retention) are usually *pranayama* practices that all can practice safely and can be substituted if *Kabbalabhati* (shining skull breath exercise) isn't a safe option, which is usually practiced in a Sivananda Yoga class. Mental repetition of a mantra while focusing on the breath (in sync with the breath) can also be done during any part of the practice.

Photo below: Full Yogic Breath

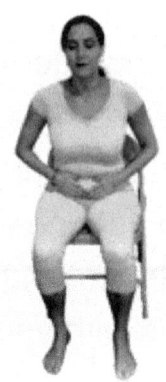

*Photo below: Alt. Nostril Breath with the Palms
Flat, Anuloma Viloma*

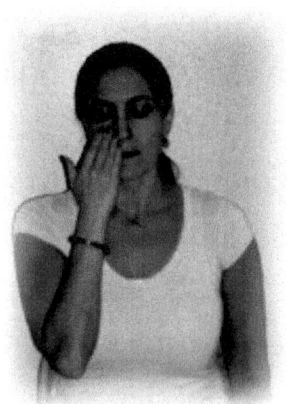

For details on how to practice Alternate Nostril Breath, see the Breathing Exercises chapter in this book.

Warm-ups

See the Sun Salutations previously taught in this book, with Seated and Standing Chair Yoga Sun Salutation options, for the adaptions to the Sun Salutations, *Surya Namaskar,* or see the images on the following pages for ideas how to adapt.

You may need a chair for only one or two of the postures in the Sun Salutation, but not for all. For example, a standing Chair Yoga Sun Salutation example of "Inverted V" pose (Downward Facing Dog) can be modified if you can't comfortably put weight on the wrists or knees, or if you have vertigo and can not put your head fully down. In that case, you can practice the Sun Salutations on the yoga mat with a chair out in front, as in the photos on the next page, for the one or two poses that the chair will be needed. However, you may not need a chair for all of the postures in the Sun Salutations. If you do, try the Standing Chair Yoga Sun Salutation or Seated versions, as in the following pages.

An example is the Standing Chair Yoga "Inverted V" Pose ("Downward Facing Dog, *Adho Mukha Svanasana*). Below is an adaption of the posture during the Sun Salutation.

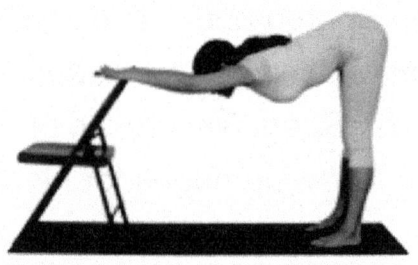

Another example the Standing Chair Yoga Lunge Pose during Sun Salutation. The photo below demonstrates using a chair back or base for support, instead of bringing the hands and back knee on the floor, along side the foot, as usually done in this sequence.

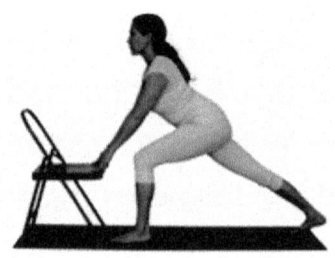

Sun Salutations *(Surya Namaskar)*

Yoga for Everyone!

(Without chairs is in the photo below.)

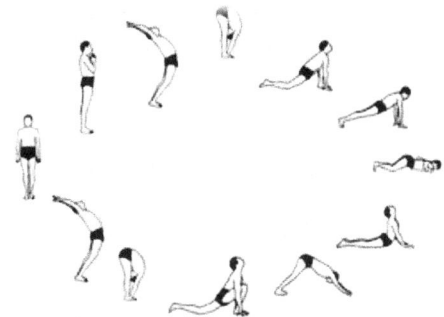

Standing Chair Yoga Sun Salutations

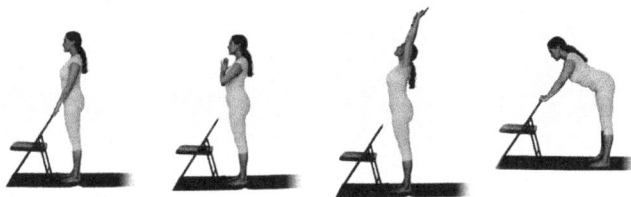

Inhale Mountain. Exhale Prayer. Inhale Arms up. Exhale Forward Bend (with the head up or resting as in the photos below).

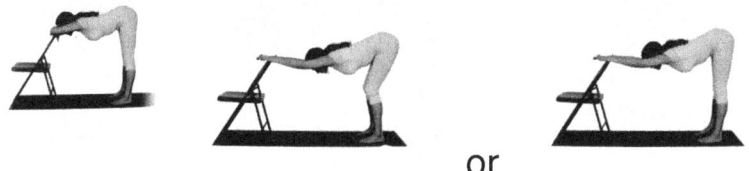

or

Forward Bend Options: The hand or head can rest on the chair top, with the knees bent or straight.

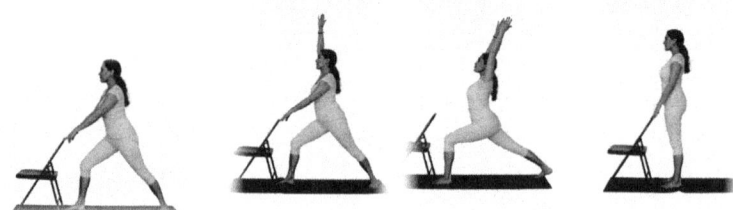

Inhale Warrior or High Lunge. Exhale relax. Inhale and lift one arm up. Exhale, lower. Inhale and lift the other arm up. Exhale, lower. Inhale and lift both arms up. Exhale, lower and step forward. Switch legs and repeat. Inhale Mountain. Exhale.

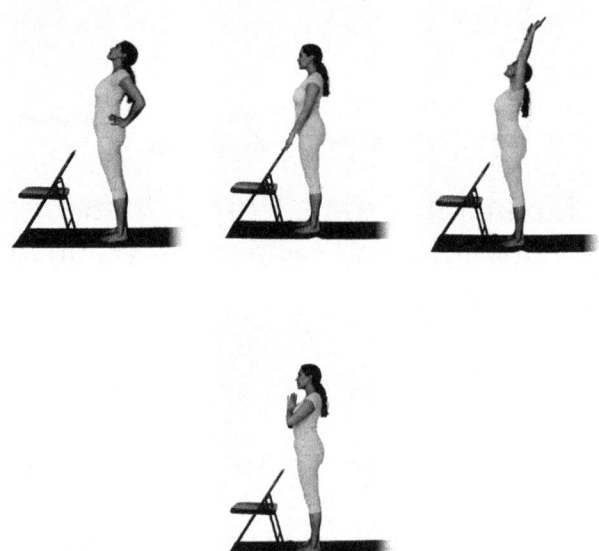

Inhale Cobra. Exhale Mountain. Inhale Arms Up. Exhale Prayer Pose. Repeat this cycle 2-8x.

Seated Sun Salutation

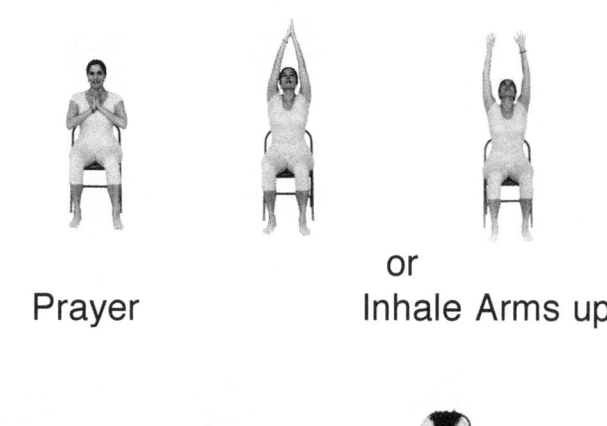

                or
Prayer   Inhale Arms up

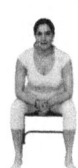 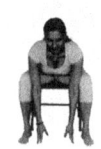 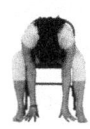

or
Exhale Forward Bend

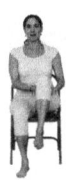 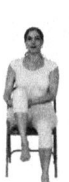

Inhale Lunge. Exhale Lower. Switch sides.

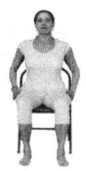 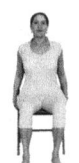 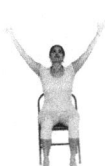 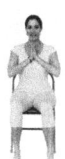

Inhale Cobra. Exhale. Inhale Arms Up. Exhale.

Repeat the Sun Salutations cycle 2-8x.

Leg Lifts

Seated Chair Yoga Alternate Leg Lifts

Keep the thighs on the chair base and lift your foot as you inhale. Exhale as you lower. Switch sides. Extend the leg and foot away from the hip joint, instead of lifting it as high as possible. Repeat 3-6 rounds.

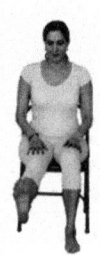 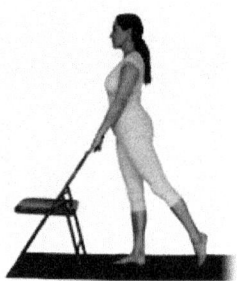

Photo (left): Seated Chair Yoga Alternate Leg Lifts
Photo (right): Standing Chair Yoga Alternate Leg Lifts

Standing Leg Lifts

Hold on to the chair top for support as you lift one leg on the inhalation. Lower the leg as you exhale. Switch sides. Repeat 4-6 rounds.

Yoga for Everyone!

Double Leg Raises

Inhale and stretch both legs out, exhale as you lower. Repeat 3-6x.

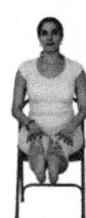 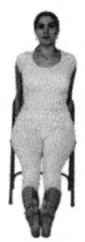

If you need more support, keep the heels on the floor (as in the photo on the bottom right, on the previous page). Inhale as you stretch the legs out. Exhale as you return to Mountain Pose.

Main *Asanas*

Headstand, *Sirshasana*

Some Chair Yoga options instead of Headstand:

1) Relaxation Pose *(Savasana)*

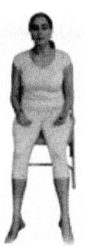

2) Cat/Cow Pose for a spinal warm up

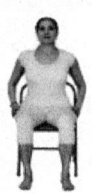
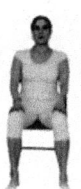

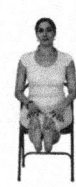

3) **Staff Pose**

4) **Standing Table Pose** with the head resting on the forearms on the chair top

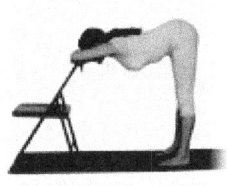

Chair Yoga Shoulderstand,
Sarvangasana

(1) Seated Elevate the legs on a second chair or (2) Legs Up on the Chair Pose, lying down. Relax and observe the breath, for 6-10 rounds.

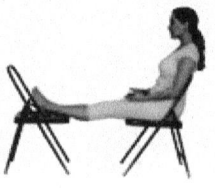

(1)

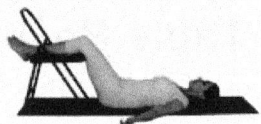

(2)

Plough, *Halasana* Chair Yoga adaptions

1) One Leg Extension: Hold the leg under one knee and extend the leg (you can use belt instead, as in the photo below). If able, hold the big toes with the index and middle finger, or hold both feet with the hands or a belt. Enjoy 5 slow deep breaths. Switch legs.

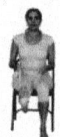

1) Or **Forward Bend** using one or two chairs *(See photos below and the on the following page.)*

Forward Bend with One Chair

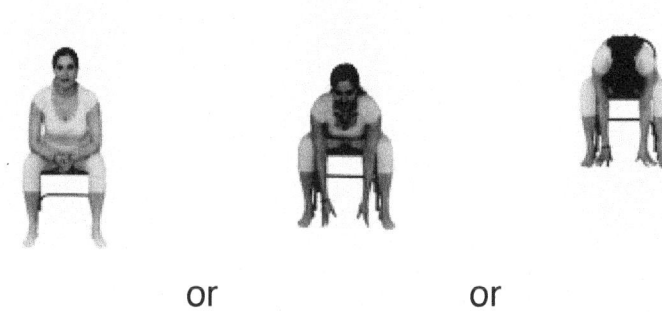

or   or

Forward Bend with Two Chairs

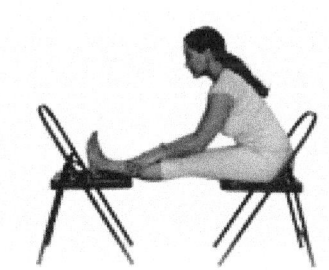

Fish, *Matsyasana*

This can be done seated or standing, using a chair for a supported backbend.

1) Interlock the fingers behind you as in the photo below. Lift the heart area and breathe.

2) If it is more comfortable, hold the bottom or back of the chair as in the photo below.

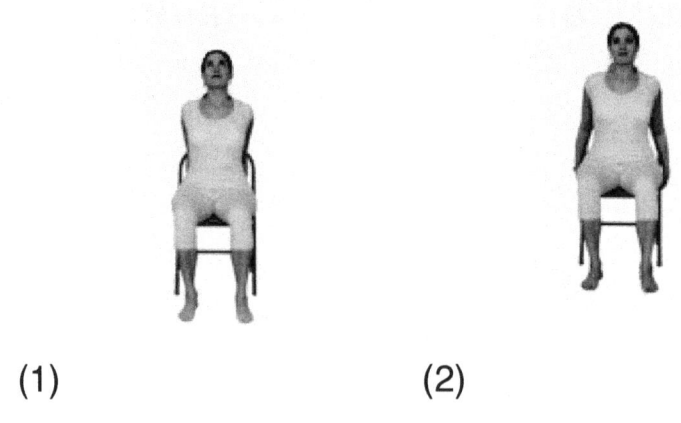

(1)   (2)

Forward Bend, *Paschimothanasana:*

1) Full or Half Seated Chair Yoga Forward Bend.

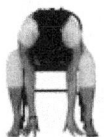
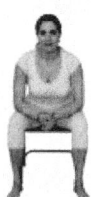

2) Or, stretch one leg out and flex the foot (photo A). Inhale as you stretch the arms up and exhale as you fold forward. Switch legs. You can also try this with both legs stretched out, keeping the buttocks firm and balanced in the chair (photo B). Place the hands on the side or back of the chair base for support. (This version is not as stable as the one leg stretched version.)

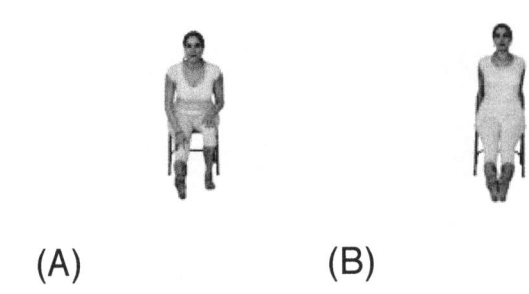

(A)   (B)

3) Or you can use a second chair for a full leg extension, as in the photo below.

Using Two Chairs

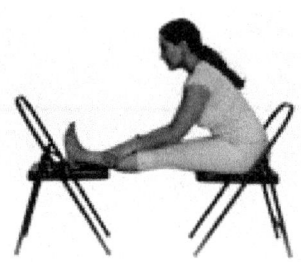

Cobra, *Bhujangasana:* Seated and standing

This may also be helpful for those in the second or third trimester of pregnancy or for those who are not able to lie on the floor (from an injury or post surgery, etc.)

1) Place the hands on the hips or thighs as you lift the heart. Keep the tailbone down and navel in towards the spine (neutral pelvis, not overarching the low back). Move the elbows towards each other. Breathe and hold the pose or go in and out of the pose gently a few times with the breath. See the photos on the following page.

Seated Cobra, *Bhujangasana*

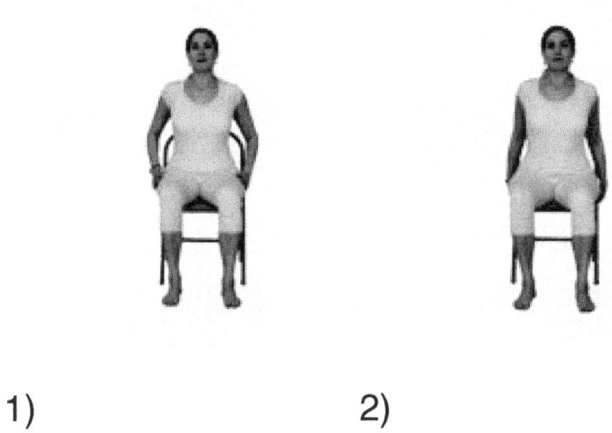

1)   2)

2) Bring the hands to the back of the chair base or to the back of the chair back/chair arms. Breathe. Lift the heart area and feel the rib area opening.

3) Interlock the fingers behind the back. Lift the heart area as the arms pull back & down.

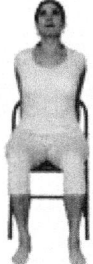

3)

Standing Cobra: Keep the tailbone moving down and the navel area in towards the spine (to lengthen and stabilize the low back).

1) Interlock the fingers behind you and stretch the hands towards the floor.

2) For more low back support, place the hands on the lower back, as in the photo below.

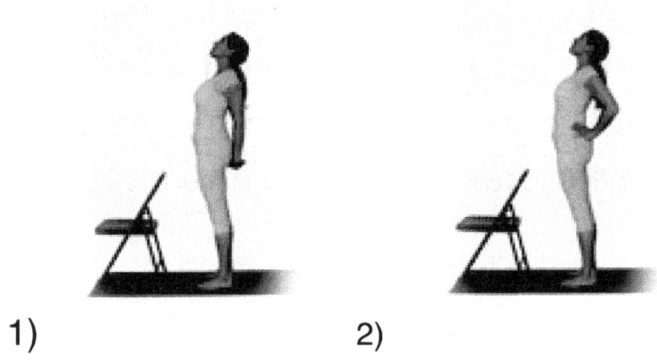

1)   2)

Half Locust, *Ardha Salabhasana*

Stand behind the chair and hold the chair back. Lift and extend one leg and hold. Keep the tailbone down, so that there is no strain or overarching of the low back. If able, you can take one hand off the chair, or both and balance. This is also a prenatal variation of the posture. See the photo on the following page.

Yoga for Everyone!

Half Locust, *Ardha Salabhasana*

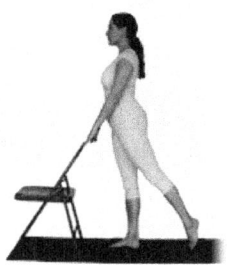

Standing Half Bow, *Ardha Dhanurasana*

Bring the hands to the low back/hip area. Inhale as you lift the chest bone (sternum). Hold onto the left foot with the left hand. Hold onto your pants or use a yoga belt if you don't reach the foot. You can also lift the foot up and place the hand on the hip, if holding the foot or belt is not accessible. Switch sides and hold as long as comfortable. (See the Cosmic Dancer Pose in Balance Poses)

Seated Half Bow Variation, *Ardha Dhanurasana*

If the chair has open sides as in the photo below, you can turn the body to the side so that both legs and feet are on one the side of the chair, with the side body (waist) facing the chair back.

Then, if able, hold onto the outside foot with the outside hand (the hand and foot furthest away from the chair back). Hold onto your pants or use a yoga belt if needed. You can also lift the foot up and place the hand on the hip if holding the foot or belt is not accessible. Switch sides and hold as long as comfortable.

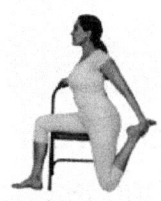

Seated Gentle Chair Yoga variation: Sitting tall, stretch the hands away from the heart for a backbend effect. Imagine you were about to hug someone and reach your arms out. Feel the heart area opening.

Spinal Twist, *Ardha Matsyendrasana*

Seated Chair Twist: Cross the legs if able, or the ankles. Inhale as you sit tall, exhale as you twist to the side (right) with the right arm to back of chair base or hanging on the outside of the chair on right side. Bring your left arm to outside of the right leg (or to the inside of left leg if needed). Hold and breathe, or go back and forth 5x in and out with breath for a more gentle practice. Example: Inhale as you relax/release to center, exhale to twist and repeat instead of holding the pose steady.

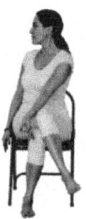 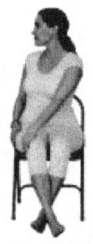

Legs crossed   Ankles crossed

Balance Poses: Crow Pose, *Bakasana*

Place your hands on the chair arms (if the chair does not have arms, as in the photo below you can place the hands onto the chair base) and try to lift the spine or lift the body if the chair. This creates a similar work in the core, strengthening the abdominals as in the balancing **Crow Pose**. See the photo on the following page.

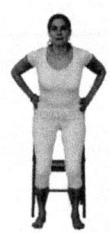

Or **Tree Pose**, *Vrkasana*

Seated versions: Lift the arms overhead, and place one heel behind the opposite ankle or inner calf. If able, place the foot on the opposite inner thigh, resting it on the chair base, as in the photos below.

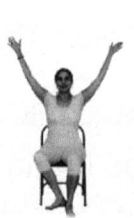 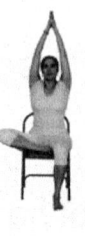

Yoga for Everyone!

Standing Tree Pose:

   Hold one hand on to the chair back for support. Lift the heel to the opposite ankle, calf, or thigh. Lift one or both arms. Focus the eyes and mind on one point in front of you. Balance.

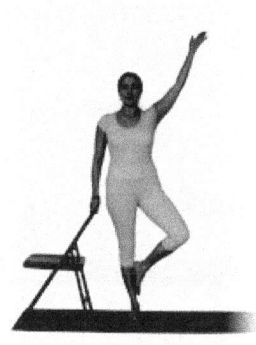

Standing Forward Bend, *Pada Hasthasana:*

   Inhale as you lift the arms up. Exhale as you fold forward. For blood pressure, vertigo (dizzy/balance issues) or other concerns or conditions, you can keep the head up and extend the spine instead. If comfortable, release the spine/head fully down and forward. You can touch the toes if able, like the full standing Forward Bend, or as in the photos, rest the head or hands on the top of the chair back. *The Seated Chair yoga Forward Bend is also an option here, as shown in the photos earlier in the sequence. For the Standing Forward Bend options, see the photo below and on the following page.

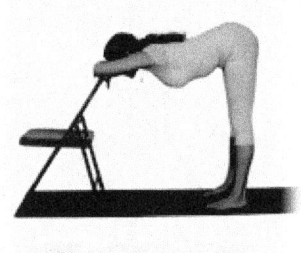

Standing Forward Bend, *Pada Hasthasana*

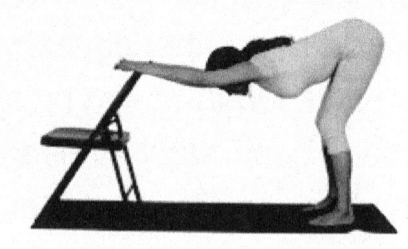

Yoga for Everyone!

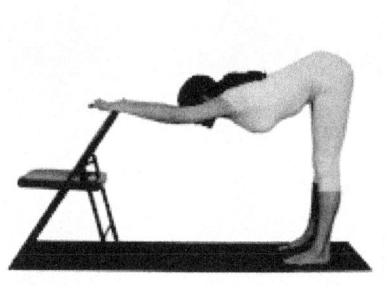

Triangle, *Trikonasana*

Seated *(Photo 1 on the following page):*
Extend the arms away from heart. Place the legs
the width of the chair base or wider. Inhale. Exhale
as you lean the upper body to one side. Switch
sides.

Standing *(Photo 2 on the following page):*
Extend the arms away from heart, placing the legs
2-3 feet wide. Inhale. Exhale as you lean the upper
body to the right side, placing the right hand on the
chair top or chair base. Stretch the left arm
towards the sky. Balance the weight equally
between both feet. Switch sides.

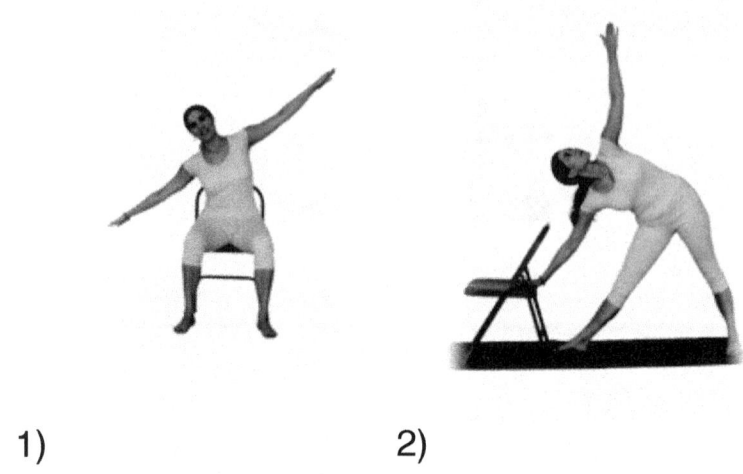

1)   2)

Chair Yoga Corpse Pose, *Savasana* for Final Relaxation

At the end of the Sivananda Yoga practice, it concludes with a long final relaxation. See the following page and the next chapter on Relaxation for more ways to practice this pose.

1) **Seated Chair Yoga Corpse Pose**: Relax in the chair. Allow the palms to rest on the thighs with the palms facing skyward. It may feel better to sit against the chair back fully, to support the low back (or use a cushion for the low back), instead of feeling compression in the low back by moving the body forward.

2) **Legs Up the Chair Pose**: Lie on the floor with the legs elevated on the chair base. Allow the hands to rest, about one foot away from the hips, with the palms facing skyward.

See the photos on the following page)

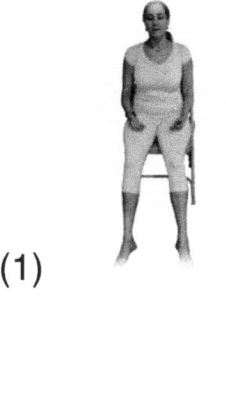

(1)

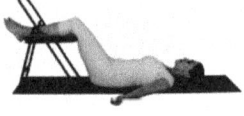

(2)

Once you are comfortable in Corpse Pose, practice the relaxation techniques below for a deeper relaxation experience.

Tense and Release Exercise

Raise the different parts of the body and squeeze, then release and relax. Start with the legs, then the arms, hips, chest and shoulders, etc. Finally squeeze the facial muscles and relax.

Autosuggestion

Beginning with the toes, feel as though a wave of relaxation is slowly moving up through the entire body. Mentally relax each toe, and then move on to the feet. Relax them completely. Say to yourself "I relax my toes, my toes are relaxed." Feel the relaxation moving up the legs. Repeat and relax up through the face, head and scalp. Finally, relax the mind. Rest in the pose for 10 minutes. 10 minutes of a deep yogic relaxation may be more restful than a full night sleep. Try it yourself and experience the benefits.

To come out of the posture, slowly sit up and sit quietly for a few minutes, chanting *Aum* or closing mantras to end the practice. If time allows, sit in silence, observing the breath and meditate.

Relaxation

5

Deep Relaxation benefits

- Relaxes the muscles
- Eases the nerves
- Calms the mind
- Relieves stress
- Brings a sense of peace

Yogic Relaxation

Corpse Pose, *Savasana*

Rest on your back. Place the legs 2-3 feet apart and the hands a few inches or more away form the hips. Let the palms face skyward. Keep the head centered over the spine. Let go of the body completely, relaxing one muscle at a time.

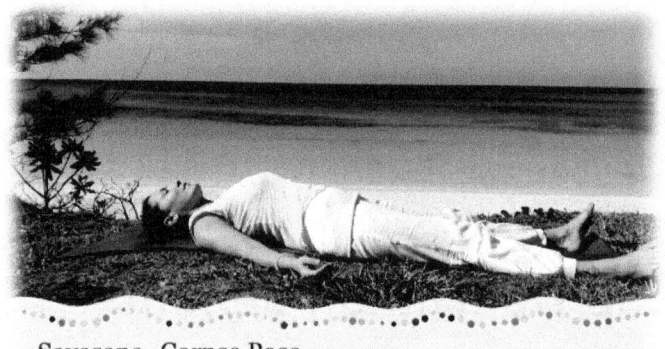

Savasana- Corpse Pose

Precautions: *For second and third trimester pregnancy adaptions, sit upright on the chair or rest on your side on the floor.

Modifications: If you have low back pain with straight legs, see the following pages for adaptions, bending the knees, or using a rolled blanket under the knees.

Final Relaxation

After each session of practicing the yoga exercises, postures and/or breath work, it is best to relax for 5 to15 minutes or more. Enjoy this time to integrate the physical postures and practice you just completed. To receive the maximum benefits of the yoga practice, stay awake, although deeply relaxed so that you can observe the relaxation process.

Gentle Yoga Corpse Pose, *Savasana*

Lying on your back, bend the knees and place the feet wider than hip width apart, about the width of your yoga mat. Rest the knees against each other or place a rolled towel or blanket under the knees (see the photos on the following page). Relax the legs, the back, the shoulders and the entire body.

Photo below: Lying on the Back with Knees Bent

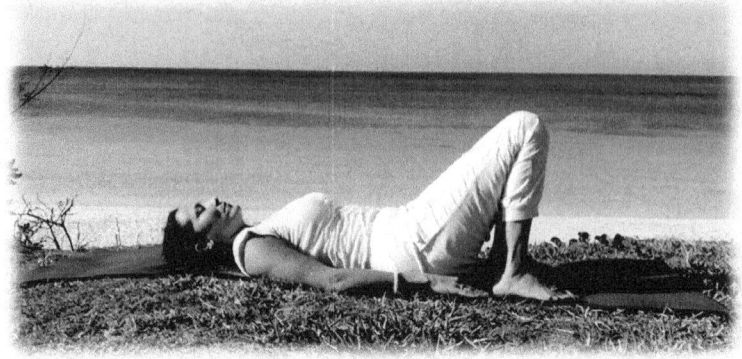

Photo below: Place a rolled blanket, towel or yoga bolster under the knees.

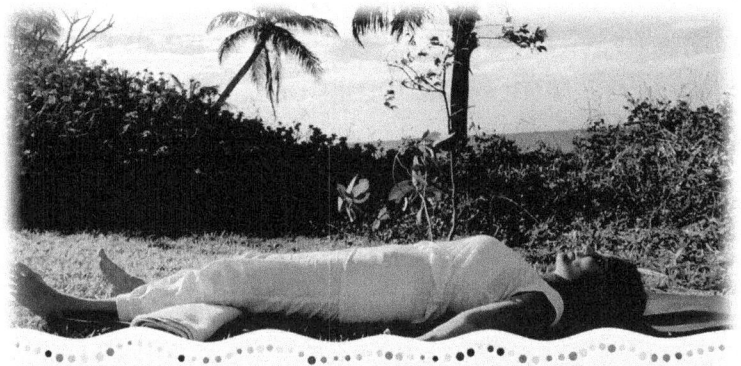

Savasana (Corpse Pose) with the knees supported

Benefits: Calms the nerves and the mind and relaxes the entire body. This variation is useful for those with low back pain, injuries or low back discomfort.

Chair Yoga Corpse Pose, *Savasana*

Sitting in a chair, rest against the chair back. You can place pillows, blankets or a yoga mat behind your low back or along your spine. You can also sit upright (instead of collapsing the low back). The palms face up as they rest on the thighs or the arms can rest along side the chair with the palms facing forward or up. Relax and enjoy the benefits of your practice. Rest and relax the muscles, rest the nerves and calm the mind.

Benefits: This Chair Yoga version is useful to take a few minute relaxation break at work, while traveling or on a lunch break (it can be done on a park bench.) This is also useful while waiting for a doctor appointment or any place where you need to calm the mind and the nerves.

Chair Yoga Final Relaxation

Sitting in a chair, rest the hands on the thighs with the palms facing up and the back resting against the chair. Tense & release each muscle, then practice autosuggestion silently repeating, "I relax my feet, my feet relax" for each part of the body. Observe the body relaxing then observe the breath for 5-10 minutes. See the photo on the following page, followed by other Chair Yoga relaxation pose options, including Legs Up the Chair Pose and elevating the legs on a second chair.

Seated Relaxation Pose

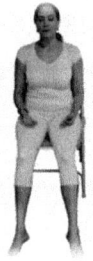

Legs up the Chair

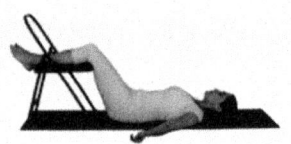

Two Chairs with Legs Elevated

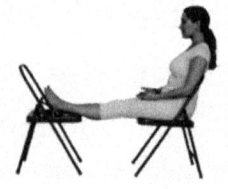

Yoga for Everyone!

Relaxation Techniques

Tense and Release

Tense and release each muscle in the body to feel the difference between tension and relaxation. Raise the different parts of the body and squeeze, then release and relax. Start with the legs, then the arms, hips, chest and shoulders, etc. Finally squeeze the facial muscles and relax.

Autosuggestion

Then you can practice "autosuggestion" by mentally repeating, "I relax my toes, my toes relax", as you bring awareness to the toes. Mentally relax each toe, and then move on to the feet. Feel the feet relax from deep within. Then shift the awareness to the ankles as you repeat silently, "I relax my ankles, my ankles relax." Repeat with the knees, legs, low back, hips, middle back, upper back, stomach, digestive organs, heart, lungs, shoulders, arms, elbows, wrists, hands, fingers, neck, throat, jaw, eyes, scalp and ears (in this order). Finally, relax mind. Rest in complete silence for 5 to 15 minutes or as needed.

To come out Corpse Pose, slowly move the

fingers and toes and roll to the right side. Slowly sit up and sit quietly for a few minutes in meditation seat (sitting tall in a chair or cross-legged). Chant Om 3x or other closing *mantras* to complete the practice.

Additional Visualization techniques:

You can then visualize you are lying on your favorite beach. As you observe the breath, feel as if waves of relaxation are entering the body with each inhale. Exhale as you relax. Ease out of the posture slowly and sit upright. Meditate on the breath for a few minutes.

Benefits: Final Relaxation in *Savasana* relaxes the physical body, nervous system and the mind. This gives us time to integrate the physical exercises and breathing practices. It stimulates the parasympathetic nervous system for calming, restoring energy and healing. This is especially helpful when recovering from injuries, chronic illness or post-traumatic stress. It is. useful in general for all to do daily, to ease the nerves from ongoing stress.

Closing Chants/Mantras/Prayers:

Repeat out loud or silently:

Om shanti, shanti, shanti

Om peace, peace, peace.

Add other mantras, uplifting prayers or songs that you may resonate with, to bring feelings of joy and deep inner peace. Feel the peace of your true essence and union with your innermost Self. That is yoga.

Ancient prayer for knowing our inner, true Self:

Asato Ma Sat Gamaya

Lead us from the unreal to the real.

Tamasoma Jyotir Gamaya

Lead us from darkness to light.

Mrityor Maamritam Gamaya

Lead us from fear of death/anxiety,

To knowledge of our eternal soul.

Aum. Shanti, Shanti, Shanti-e Peace. Peace. Peace.

"Some people might think that by practicing Yoga you're running away from the world and are not going to enjoy anything. But yogis are the people who are going to enjoy everything. Because when you're the master of your life, you're not controlled by anything and you can enjoy everything. This is the aim of Yoga." -Swami Satchidananda

"Individual Peace paves the way for world peace. The attainment of inner calm is the greatest work you can do for humanity." Sivananada

"The cause of *bandha* and moksha (bondage and liberation) is our own minds. If we think we are bound, we are bound. If we think we are liberated, we are liberated . . . . It is only when we transcend the mind that we are free from all these troubles. (117)"
— Swami Satchidananda, The Yoga Sutras

Yoga at Work

6

In Chapter 6, Yoga at Work

- Yoga works at work!
- 1-5 minute yoga breaks
- Eye exercises
- Shoulder exercises
- 2-5 minute meditations

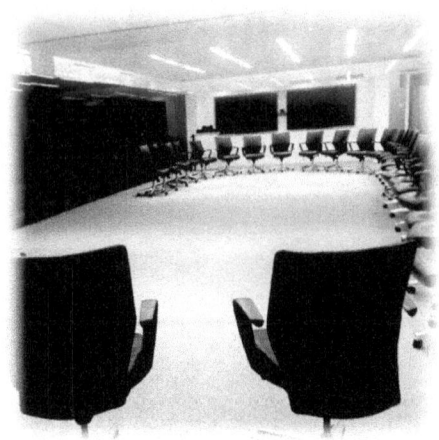

"Yoga works at work" is my motto for offering yoga at the work place. You can do yoga at your desk, at work or at home, to decrease tension, avoid repetitive stress injuries, to ease neck, shoulder and back pain, to ease blurry vision syndrome from extensive computer use and to keep focused and refreshed during the work day. You can practice yoga without having to change into workout clothes or leave your desk. Chair Yoga makes it accessible and enjoyable to practice yoga, even during the busy workday.

Particularly good are the neck, shoulder and wrist exercises. However, all are equally beneficial to keep the body flexible and relaxed.

Here is an example of a short work break you can take:

3 minute Shoulder and Neck Release sequence

Take three slow, deep breaths. Feel yourself relax. Inhale as you shrug (slide) your shoulders up to the ears. Exhale as you drop and lower them. Repeat 3 to 6x. Imagine all of your tensions and worries leaving you with each exhalation.

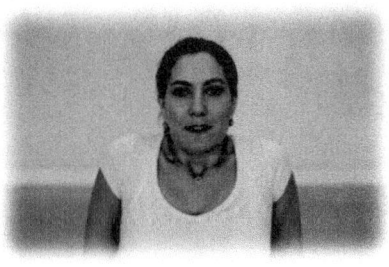

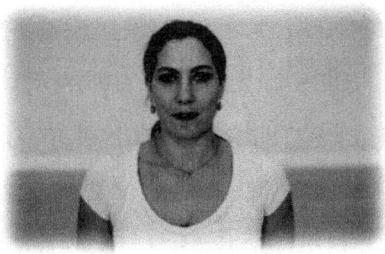

Benefits: Eases neck and shoulder tensions. Reminds the shoulders and upper back muscles to relax while on the computer or from general stress.

The Shoulder Shrugs are also helpful to remind the neck and shoulders to relax on airplanes, on long road trips, during conferences or during long work meetings.

Photo below: Chair Yoga at your desk

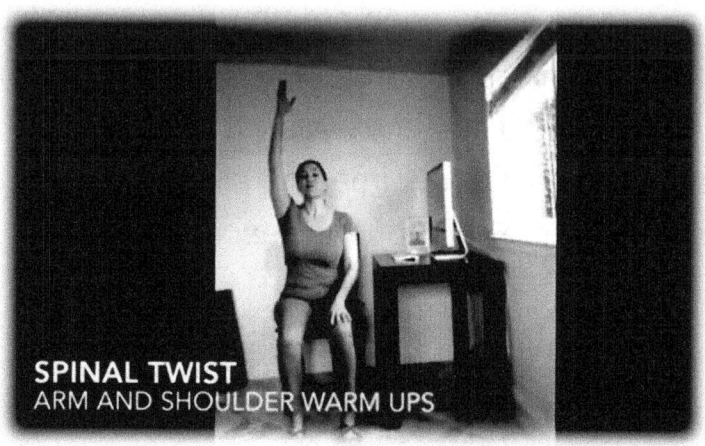

SPINAL TWIST
ARM AND SHOULDER WARM UPS

Simple Breath Awareness Exercise

To calm the mind, start to observe your breath. It may be easier to focus if you close your eyes. If you are at your desk, turn away from the computer screen. This is a simple exercise to practice anywhere and anytime. Start with 2 minutes a day and build up to 10 minutes a day twice a day. This will calm the mind and ease the nerves, allowing you to go back to work with improved concentration and clarity.

Eye Exercises, *Netra Vyayam*

Here are some old, traditional yoga exercises for the eyes, specifically helpful in the modern era to ease computer-related vision issues, including getting dry and irritated or blurry eyes from long hours looking at the computer screen. Sit tall in the chair, keeping the breath relaxed and rhythmic. Try not to move the head during the eye exercises.

- Roll the eyes up and down. Repeat 5x.
- Roll the eyes right to left. Repeat 5x.

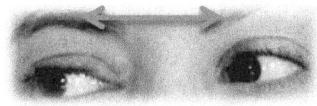

- Roll the eyes to the upper right corner, then to the lower left. Repeat 5x. Switch directions. Roll the eyes to the upper left corner, then to the lower right corner.

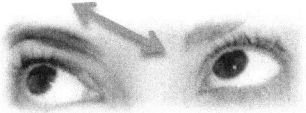

- Roll the eyes in circles clockwise. Try to even out the movement as best you can. Repeat 3 to 5x. Reverse the direction, circling the eyes counterclockwise.

One-Minute Meditation for Stress Relief

Sit in a comfortable position with the spine tall but not tense. Feel your feet on the floor. Support the low back with a pillow if needed. Close your eyes. Bring yourself into the present moment. Become aware of your body and surroundings. Take a few deep sighs. Observe then regulate the breath with rhythmic, deep and slow breathing. Allow the mind to wander at first. Focus at the brow point (between the eyebrows), the navel or the heart center where the mind can rest. When the mind drifts, bring it back to the breath, which takes you back to the present moment.

Start with one minute a day for a week. Even if your mind isn't calm during the meditation, you will see the effects after daily practice. Increase this as time goes on to 3 minutes, then 5 minutes. You can do this at your desk in a chair, or in the mornings or evenings in a quiet place at home. Be regular in your 1 to 5 minute meditation practice for the best results. At home or during long lunch breaks, try building up to 10-30 minutes a day. Meditation brings a sense of clarity, creativity and deep inner peace.

Yogic Diet

7

In Chapter 7, Yogic Diet

Yogic Diet
- Includes vegetables, fruits and whole grains
- Is well balanced
- Is healthy and delicious
- Brings radiant health
- Does not harm animals
- Is ideal for meditation

Yogic Diet

Yoga exercises, breathing practices, relaxation, meditation and mantras are all helpful to create a more balanced and healthy body and a peaceful mind. What we put into our bodies is just as important as the other aspects of the yoga lifestyle. Maybe even more so because of the fact that we eat every day and multiple times a day.

Shifting to or keeping a vegetarian (no meat or fish) or vegan diet (no meat, fish or dairy) to help create a healthier body and a more peaceful mind can be a very simple process. Just as we brush our teeth and shower to keep our body clean, often without much thought, so we can eat foods that keep us clean and nourish us on the inside as well, all while not harming ourselves, the environment or animals in the process.

The Yoga Sutras of Patanjali says that *Ahimsa* (non-violence) is the first principle in the philosophy of yoga, establishing a base to keep the physical body healthy and the mind less agitated. Verse 2.35 that mentions this, in Sanskrit states that *ahimsapratishthayam tatsannidhau vairatyagah,* which means that when a yogi becomes firmly established in non-violence *(ahimsa),* other people around him (or her) will give up aggression or hostility.

Most of the yoga masters teach that it is difficult to control your mind when you are eating meat (there are scientific reasons for this, including the adrenalin and hormones associated with the way the animals are raised and slaughtered, among others). All of the myths and debates about why one needs meat have been disproven in this modern age, and in fact it has been shown that vegetarian diet is healthier.

Yogic diet is a vegetarian diet, one in which vegetables, fruits, nuts, grains and dairy are eaten in balance to create optimal health and vitality. However, now, because of the violence in factory farming (which account for 99% of animals and animal products eaten in USA per the Factory Farm Awareness Coalition facts), most true yogis are shifting, or have shifted to a vegan diet, which does not include dairy (no cheese, milk or butter). In the modern age there are so many substitutes such as soy, rice, hemp or coconut milk or cashew based butters, that it is now very simple to shift to be vegan, at least for those with health food stores in their area or the willingness to educate themselves on how to shift to this simple diet. Many who have become vegan have reported having chronic illness and ailments disappear as well as weight loss, increased sense of well-being and improved energy.

With the proper balance of the protein and nutrients your body needs, you can feel more energy and vitality. Human beings do not need any animal products to live healthy. I am a living example, as I have never eaten animals, being raised vegetarian since birth, thanks to the yogis and my parents who learned from them.

Keeping it simple, not eating too much or too little protein and balancing our meals with vegetables, grains and protein, while making it appealing to yourself, creates a diet that is "easeful, useful, and peaceful", as Swami Satchidananda used to say that yoga (and life) should be.

Ahimsa is the Sanskrit term for "non-violence", the basis of the yogic living, according to the Yoga Sutras of Patanjali. So does this include the animals? Yogic philosophy believes in not harming, that is clear. And yes, this does include the animals. This is why the yogis were vegetarian.

In the Yoga Sutras, *ahimsa*, is apart of the

yamas (ethical observances) the first limb of 8 limbs of yoga, steps to achieve final liberation, bliss consciousness (s*amadhi).* The third of 8 limbs, yoga *asana* (yoga posture), is more commonly practiced as the focus at most modern yoga studios and health clubs. However, as Dharma Mitra, yoga master in NYC reminds us (in a light hearted way), "Yoga without the *Yamas* is like spaghetti without the sauce. More seriously, as Mahatma Gandhi, said "The most violent weapon on earth is the table fork." Dharma Mittra has also said "that one must extend one's compassion beyond one's pets" and that "when one eats animals one is engaging in cruelty." In Sri Dharma's words, "Without taking on the *yama* of *ahimsa,* there is little benefit to observing the other four *yamas* or any other aspect of the holy science of yoga."

I personally feel blessed to have been raised vegetarian, thanks to the yogis. My mother and father became full vegetarian after learning its health and non-violence benefits from the Gurus. They ate no meat, poultry, or fish by the time I was born, so I was also raised vegetarian and I have never tasted meat or fish in my life. I simply don't see dead animals as food. Instead I see animals as intelligent, sentient beings, that feel pain and want to live, just like us.

More recently though, I also learned the harm done to animals in the dairy industry, including killing innocent chicks and baby cows (who can't produce eggs or milk), are also killed (calves they then call 'veal'). I visited the Animal Place Rescue Farm in Grass Valley, CA, and saw for myself the small veal crates that so cruelly hold baby cows captive for a few weeks, where they can not even turn around, let alone nurse on their mother, and then are slaughtered for people's food choices, all because the male baby cows don't produce milk, which is profit for the dairy industry. Is human profit worth the suffering and life of another living creature? Not to me. When I learned that the dairy industry is tied into the meat industry I realized I was still supporting and ingesting violence by eating eggs, cheese and drinking cow's milk. Many yoga ashrams now have vegan options, as even the yogic diet is shifting with the times, to be more sustainable and adhere to ahimsa.

According to the Factory Farm Awareness Coalition, 99 percent of animal products come from factory farms. They also say that 'even in cage free operations, most chickens see sunlight for the first time when taken to slaughter." There is no way to deny the violence in consuming animals; with proper education the facts are clear. This is not *ahimsa*, and creates an unfathomable amount of suffering to living, breathing beings. Yoga Master Sivananda said "People who are slaves to the flesh-eating habit cannot give up animal diet, because they have become confirmed and inveterate meat-eaters, and hence they try to justify their habit by various arguments and statistics. One cannot change their ways merely by argumentation and disputation. Ultimately, it is only the force of personal example that has a strong effect upon the people around you." - Sivananda, Bliss Divine Yoga- Vedanta Forest Academy, Divine Life Society; 1st edition (1964) With education, awareness and willingness, we can all take compassion off the yoga mat, and onto our plates.

Shifting to a compassionate way of eating does not have to be hard. There are amazing organizations doing great work to educate the masses on how to live healthy and support the least mount of harm done to animals and the earth by going vegan. Mercy for Animals and PETA are two of those that even provide vegan starter kids and a plethora of online recipes and videos for ideas.

Yoga Masters Dharma Mittra and Sharon Gannon of Jivamukti yoga, both in NYC, are advocates of needing to go vegan in order to live a true yogic and compassionate lifestyle. Dharma Mittra says "If you are interested to go deeper into yoga, you should read The Yoga-Sutras and The Hatha Yoga Pradipika. For those just interested in living a more ethical life, there's The Dammapada." He also says "The action of compassion is to see yourself in others." In that text the Dammapada, the Buddha said "All beings tremble before violence. All fear death. All love life. See yourself in others. Then whom can you hurt? What harm can you do?" Dhammapada 129- 130

Sharon Gannon, who wrote Yoga and Vegetarianism says "By enslaving other animals and abusing them through lifelong torture, degradation and eventual slaughter, we deprive them of freedom and happiness. How can we ourselves hope to be free or happy when our own lives are rooted in depriving others of the very thing we say we value most in life – the freedom to pursue happiness? If you want to bring more peace and happiness into your own life, the method is to stop causing violence and unhappiness in the lives of others. We cannot demand something that we ourselves are not willing to embody.

Through the practice of yoga and veganism, we can realize that we were meant to live in harmony with all the other animals and all of life. We come to know that our physical bodies function better without having to instill fear into others and to kill them, and that there is no nutrient that we need that we can't get directly from plant sources or from sunlight. We come to recognize that our old bodies can be transformed and become light and whole – holy bodies, used as vehicles to bring peace. The fork can be a powerful weapon of mass-destruction or a tool to lead a movement of peaceful coexistence. Eating a compassionate vegan diet will stop war, create peace in one's body, peace with the animal nations, and peace on Earth." -Sharon Gannon, adapted from Yoga and Vegetarianism

Reducing suffering and having compassion for all living beings is my focus as a yoga teacher and student and spiritual practitioner. It happens to also prevent disease, increase vitality and helps the earth.

It seems many are now "going green" by recycling more and being more mindful of eating organic foods and such. In fact, the most support one can offer Mother Earth is to eat less or no meat. "You save more water by not eating a pound of meat than you do by not showering for six months!" as calculated by PETA (www.peta.org).

This is true because Agriculture is responsible for 80 to 90% of US water consumption per the USDA ERS. It was also found that 2,500 gallons of water are used to make one pound of US beef (from Dr. George Borgstrom, Chairman of Food Science and Human Nutrition Dept of College of Agriculture and Natural Resources, Michigan State University).

Consider this as well: "animal agriculture is responsible for up to 91% of Amazon destruction." For more facts and information such as this you can see the documentary Cowspiracy: the Sustainability Secret.

For myself, what is most important is to not harm innocent living beings that love and nurture their young, fear and tremble in pain and want to live and enjoy life, as us humans. The health and environmental reasons are also meaningful and important but I personally would not want to eat an animal that was harmed and then kill. For the sake of my animal friends, I am supportive of anyone wanting to shift to more compassionate eating and living. I am a voice for the animals and do hope humanity learns to live in a harmony with all of the earth's inhabitants in this modern age.

To conclude, I will share the excerpts from the yoga master Sivananda's book Bliss Divine (1964 first edition). And as Sivananda said "May you shine as a dynamic Yogi by the practice of selfless service! May you enjoy the true bliss of the eternal."

"If you want to stop taking mutton, fish, etc., just see with your own eyes the pitiable, struggling condition of the animals at the time of killing. Now mercy and sympathy will arise in your heart. You will determine to give up flesh-eating. If you fail in this attempt, just change your environment and live in a vegetarian hotel where you cannot get mutton and fish, and move in that society where there is only vegetable diet. Always think of the evils of flesh-eating and the benefits of a vegetarian diet. If this also cannot give you sufficient strength to stop this habit, go to the slaughter- house and the butcher's shop and personally see the disgusting, rotten muscles, intestines, kidneys and other nasty parts of the animals which emits bad smell. This will induce

Vairagya (dispassion) in you and a strong disgust and hatred for meat-eating.

All slaughter-houses should be abolished, and the use of animal flesh as food should be absolutely given up. Flesh-eating is unnecessary, unnatural, and unwholesome. The countless instances of reputed philosophers, authors, scholars, athletes, saints, Yogins, Rishis who lived on vegetable diet conclusively prove that vegetarian diet produces supreme powers both of mind and body, and is highly conducive for divine contemplation and practice of Yoga.

Man is created a frugivorous or fruit-eating creature. This scientific fact is evident on a comparison with the carnivorous animals from whom he differs completely in respect of his internal organs, teeth, and external appearances, whereas, anatomically, he is most intimately allied to the anthropoid apes whose diet consists of fruits, cereals, and nuts.

When man abandons flesh foods and takes his nutrient direct from nature's hand, of well-ripe and healthy fruits and grains, nuts and vegetables with addition of honey, cheese and milk, we shall find a large number of diseases disappearing.

People will have more power of endurance and attain longevity.

What is needed is a well-balanced diet, not a rich diet. A rich diet produces diseases of the liver, kidneys, and pancreas. A well-balanced diet helps a man to grow, to turn out more work, increases his body-weight, and keeps up efficiency, stamina, and a high standard of vim and vigor. " -Sivananda

For more on Ahimsa: nonviolent eating and living, I have an ebook and book on this topic, pictured below. You can also view daily posts on vegan recipes and animal rights current news on my pages: www.facebook.com/ahimsadiet and www.twitter.com/ahimsadiet

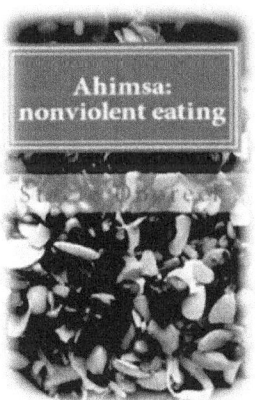 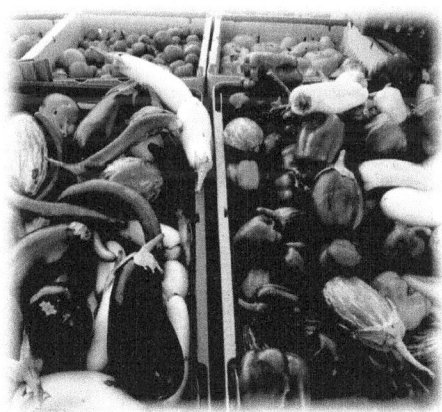

Vegan Dogs

Did you know that dogs can be vegan too? To help the earth's sustainability and not contribute to violence, even your dog can be a yogi (and a vegan). After all, the dogs already do the yoga postures which we learned rom them (Downward Facing Dog). There are several vegan dog food companies now to help this mission of *ahimsa,* non-violence. My father's dog has been vegan for a long time is extremely healthy. Davinchi, my father's vegan standard poodle is pictured below.

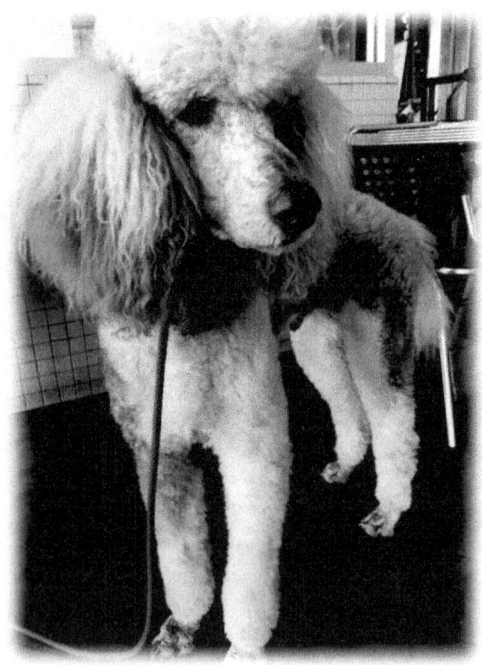

Cows are my friends, not food. The photo below is of Panda the cow. Panda was rescued and is now living free at the Animal Place in Grass Valley, California. I love to visit the animals here when I go to the Sivananda Yoga Farm near by. All animals deserve freedom and to live in peace, just like us. Yogic diet promotes harmony with the animals, the earth and all living beings.

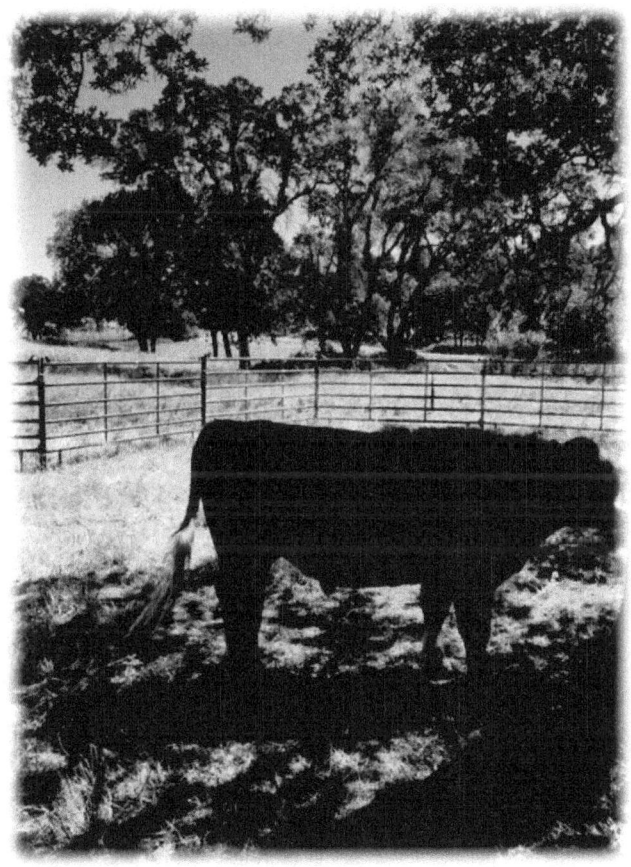

Recipes

Enjoy this recipe for its protein, with steamed greens and/or salad for a healthy and simple meal. Note: You can also shave some fresh ginger to put on top before baking, and if you are vegan, substitute the butter with oil or vegan butter, to coat the pan and put tamari on top of the tofu.

This is from the Sivananda Yoga Cookbook:

BAKED TOFU RECIPE *(vegan version)*

Serves 4

Ingredients:

1lb. tofu, Vegan butter (cashew based, for example), Tamari, Good-tasting yeast

Instructions:

Slice the tofu into 10 to 12 slices. Melt vegan butter in a saucepan and add tamari for flavor. Layer the tofu in a cookie sheet or large pan and then pour the vegan butter-tamari mixture over it. Sprinkle some yeast on top of the tofu, and bake in the oven at 375 degrees Fahrenheit for 20 minutes or until the tofu is lightly roasted and crispy.

Another recipe from the Sivananda Yoga Cookbook and ashrams:

SUNFLOWER SEED DRESSING

This is the most popular salad dressing in the Sivananda Yoga ashrams worldwide. Try some on your leafy greens!

Blend 1 C oil, 1/2 C tamari, 1/2 C lemon juice and 1 to 2 C sunflower seeds until you get a smooth and creamy consistency. If the consistency is too thick, add some water; if too thin, add more sunflower seeds. To this mixture, you can add any herb or spice you prefer. Taste and adjust. Makes 4-5 cups.

STACIE'S KALE CHIPS

For a healthy snack at home or work, try kale chips. This is a healthy alternative to potato chips.

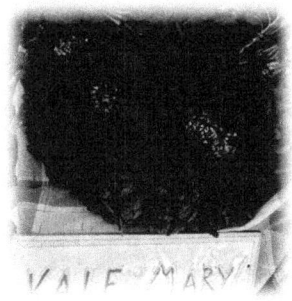

Preheat the oven to 360-370 degrees. Put coconut oil in a pan. Bake small pieces of kale broken up (or cut up) at 370 degrees Fahrenheit, with coconut oil and salt and pepper (optional) lightly sprinkled on before baking. You can also bake it with Nutritional Yeast (high in B-12 so is great for vegans). Bake 15-20 minutes.

Ahimsa: Non-Violent Eating Book Recipes

EDAMAME & POMEGRANATE SEED SALAD

Ingredients: Edamame, sliced almonds, pomegranate seeds, cucumbers, carrots, sprouted mung beans with black pepper, fresh organic lemon juice and olive oil

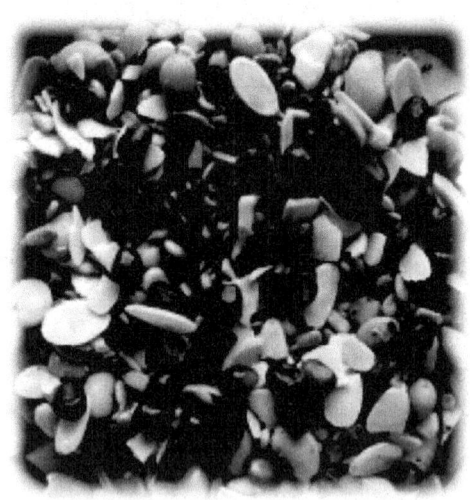

POWER PROTEIN SPROUTED LENTIL SALAD

Soak lentils over night (you can also sprout them for an extra day), sliced almonds, sesame seeds, parsley flakes (or add fresh organic greens). Add some oil and fresh squeezed lemon. This is simple and nutritious!

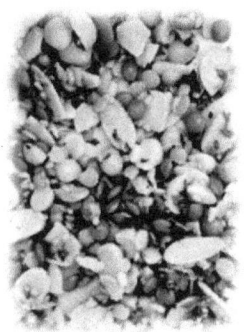

STACIES TRAIL MIX

Ingredients: Organic raisins, goji berries, sunflower seeds, roasted edamame and pistachio nuts

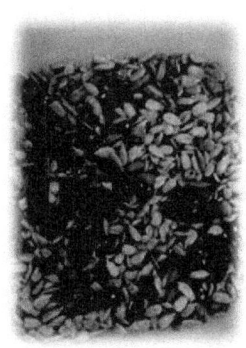

VEGAN VEGETABLE LASAGNA

Boil lasagna flat noodles. Bake or sauté a few vegetables (for example: organic spinach, organic zucchini thinly sliced and baked organic sliced mushrooms). Layer the noodles with tomato sauce and vegetables and bake it with the vegan cheese below, at 365 degrees for 30 minutes or as needed.

A vegan substitute for ricotta cheese is:

Ingredients: Blended tofu, Organic fresh lemon juice, Garlic, Nutritional yeast (*high in B-12 vitamins so is great for vegans!), Salt and pepper

Blend the ingredients above (amounts will vary for servings needed). Bake with the vegan cheese layered between the noodles, sauce and vegetables.

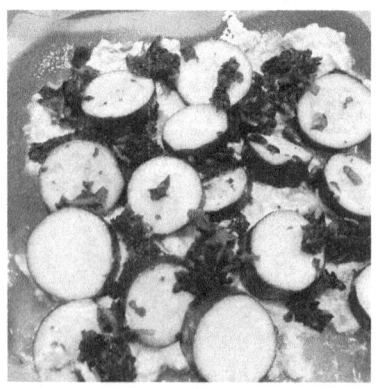

VEGAN GOLDEN MILK

Ingredients: Unsweetened Coconut, Almond or Cashew Milk, Cinnamon, Turmeric and Ginger *(Ginger is optional)*

Heat a cup of almond milk (cashew or coconut milk) until it is boiling. Mix it with a sprinkle of cinnamon and turmeric. Reduce the heat and let cool for a few minutes. Enjoy a healthy cup of Vegan Golden milk. You can also add fresh chopped ginger, which is good for your digestion.

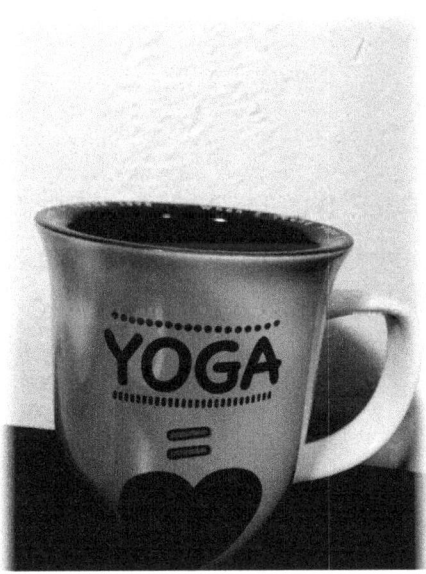

"You think a vegetable is just a food. To. me, a vegetable is as good as medicine." Yogi Bhajan

"The lion is a great meat-eater, and he is called the king of the jungle. But no animal can match the elephant, a complete vegetarian, for pure strength." Yogi Bhajan

10 tips for a Yogic lifestyle

8

In Chapter 8, Yogic Lifestyle

10 simple ideas for
- A healthy body
- A relaxed mind
- Healthy eating
- Harmonious living
- Inner peace

In modern society, there is not only a push to do more and achieve more, but a constant bombardment from media to consume more. This is taught by media images and advertisements that try to convince us that the external consumption of material things will give us greater happiness and peace of mind.

However, the truth that the yogis teach is that the way to true inner peace has nothing to do with things on the outside, nor what we accomplish, achieve and obtain—or even from what we do. Instead, the yogis teach us that being in touch with the essence of who we really are, the innermost self is the key to inner and lasting peace.

This can be realized with a few simple steps a day, practicing some simple yogic tools to connect us with our true nature. It is in this connection with the deepest part of us of that we can experience the simplicity and joy of just "being."

Swami Vishnudevananda, who founded the Sivananda Yoga centers and ashrams in the United States, said, "It is impossible to find peace outside. If you want to find peace, you have to look for peace where it is. If you want to find peace, you must first of all find it within. If you find this peace within, you will also find it outside. So if you want to have external peace, find, first of all, the peace within."

His guru, Sivananda, said, "To achieve that state of lasting happiness and absolute peace, we must first know how to calm the mind, to concentrate and go beyond the mind. By turning the mind's concentration inward, upon the self, we can deepen that experience of perfect concentration. This is the state of meditation."

To sit and do nothing but observe the breath, perhaps with a sound (mantra) or other tools to calm the mind, brings so many benefits. It is so simple that many people overlook it and seek external ways to find peace. When we start to meditate and sit still, for even a few minutes a day, we may truly see that "less is more," as joy and peace is obtained not in the "doing" but by the "being" of your true nature.

To make our lives more simple and create a few more minutes a day to meditate and "be" with our innermost self, we can follow some basic ideas from the yogic way of living.

Yoga, or "union," is an ancient science to help us reach a greater connection with ourselves and the world around us. Yoga includes postures (asanas), breathing exercises (pranayama), chanting, relaxation, meditation, nonviolent actions and diet (vegetarian), and healthy, balanced eating and living. Even trying small parts of a yogic lifestyle brings greater health and balance and can impact our life in beneficial ways.

Everyone can benefit from yoga because yoga can be modified to suit your needs. The benefits are numerous, ranging from pain relief to peace of mind.

Yoga can be summarized as a full lifestyle. Swami Vishnudevananda condensed the essence of the yoga teachings into five principles for physical and mental health, as well as spiritual growth:

Proper exercises—*asana*

Proper breathing—*pranayama*

Proper relaxation—*savasana*

Proper diet—vegetarian.

Positive thinking and meditation—*dhyana.*

Using these five principals for a holistic yogic lifestyle for inner peace, outer health, and harmony with animals and the earth, plus some additional ideas suggested here, can contribute more simplicity, more peace, and greater harmony in our day.

10 ideas that can help us simplify our lives:

Proper exercise:

Each day, do a little bit of exercise (yoga, tai chi, qigong, swimming, or walking, for example) It is better to practice yoga or tai chi 15 minutes per day than wait until your weekend or holiday schedule allows a full hour class or practice time. Modify exercise or yoga routines so that it works for your schedule. When we keep it simple, we are more likely to be consistent. Walking, tai chi, and yoga do not require any equipment and can be done anywhere.

Proper breathing:

The yogis offer breathing techniques for specific effects, such as increasing energy or calming the mind. Many practices exist, but if you just start out by simply paying attention to the breath, or even taking a few slow deep breaths a day—the most simple thing we can do without needing to change our environment—that is a great start. Also, when we slow the breath down, we activate the parasympathetic nervous system, which is the opposite of the "fight or flight" response we have when we are under stress.

Proper relaxation:

The yogis give tools for deep, conscious relaxation (often done after yoga postures), but you can even practice relaxation during a lunch break, while sitting on a bench or—if you don't have time in the day—by spending a few minutes at night being conscious of the relaxation process before you go to sleep. Simply watch the muscles in your body relax one by one as you bring awareness to each part of the body. Observe your breath, allowing the mind and body to unwind and relax deeply.

Proper diet:

The yogis have taught that there is no need to harm any living being, including the animals. A simple plant-based diet, including fruits, vegetables, legumes, and whole grains, does not

Yoga for Everyone!

harm animals or our health, and it is best for the earth. It is simple to prepare fresh salads and steamed vegetables with rice. Simple eating also is easier on the digestive tract.

Positive thinking:

It takes no time at all to change a thought. When you realize your mind is too busy or being negative, try the yogic technique *called prakti paksha bhavana* by replacing a negative thought with a positive one. Choose which thought to focus on when you meditate. "Everything that happens in your mind is reflected in your body," says the yoga master T.K.V. Desikachar.

Meditation:

Sitting in silence a few minutes or more a day allows the mind to settle and the body to relax, and that creates a better sense of well-being. Even when life is hectic and busy, allow a few minutes a day to just "be." That is so useful for the immune system, and it allows the mind to gain clarity and the body to relax and restore energy. Keep it simple. Find a quiet place in your home or outside to just pause, sit, and observe the breath. Allow the thoughts to come and go. Over time, the mind will get more quiet and peaceful.

Proper sleep:

Each day, get proper sleep and rest. The number of hours needed will vary for each person. Creating a soothing nighttime ritual may allow for deeper sleep. A nighttime ritual can include herbal tea or reading a yoga book at night instead of watching the TV or using the internet, which may create disturbances in our minds or emotions.

Unplug from technology each day:

Although cell phones, the internet, and modern technology are designed to make our lives more efficient, and even easier, they often distract us from being in the present moment, being with other people, and noticing our surroundings. Each time you go to exercise, before bedtime, or when you first wake up, try to take some time to be with your breath, body, and surroundings and take a break from computers and cell phones.

Let go of things you don't need:

A simple, zen-like environment will help the

mind focus and be more at peace. Get rid of clothes you don't need by donating them to a local homeless shelter. Donate books you no longer want. See what you can let go of to create more room for simplicity in your home, office and life. This includes not only material belongings that you no longer want or use, but excess thoughts that no longer serve your greater good and inner peace. When we let go of the old, we make room for the new.

Spend time in nature:

Nature is healing and it brings so much joy. Watching birds, feeling the sunshine on your face, and enjoying the change of seasons is so simple, yet we are often so busy in our minds that we overlook it. Physicians in San Francisco and other areas are now prescribing park time to patients. Each day, find some time to breathe in the fresh air. This can be while you walk to your car, when you're at work, or when you can take a walk through a park or on a beach. Even if you are unable to get outside, take three slow deep breaths right now and notice the trees and sky outside and come back to the present moment. Feel the body as you inhale, and relax the mind as you exhale.

Joy is within:

Go within to find joy and peace instead of finding it on the outside. It is simpler to sit a few minutes in silence, to notice the breath or enjoy a walk, than it is to need an external way to find peace. When you tap in to the peace within, it is always there to return to. Regardless of your circumstances, relationships, and outer world, the mind can always rest on the breath.

Here is a little song, called the "Yoga of Synthesis," for daily practice:

Eat a little, drink a little,

Talk a little, sleep a little,

Mix a little, move a little,

Serve a little, rest a little

Work a little, relax a little,

Do asanas a little, pranayamas a little,

Reflect a little, meditate a little,

Do Japa a little, do Kirtan a little,

Write mantras a little, have satsanga a little.

Serve, love, give, purify, meditate, realize.

Be good, do good; Be kind, be compassionate.

Enquire "Who am I?" Know the self and be free.

~ Swami Sivananda

"Awake, O Aspirant! Do vigorous *Sadhana.*
Burn all impurities. Attain illumination
through meditation." Swami Sivananda

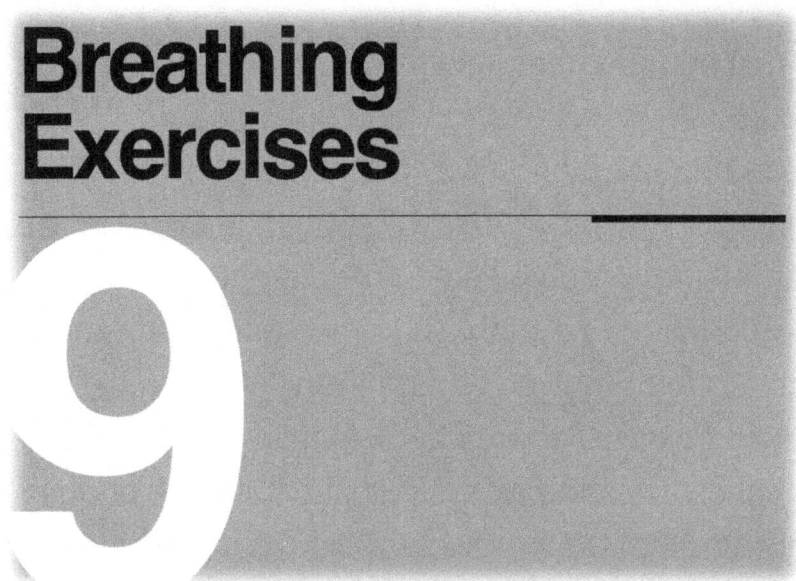

Breathing Exercises

9

In Chapter 9, Breathing Exercises

Yogic Breathing Benefits
- Calms the mind
- Relieves tension
- Helps with insomnia
- Improves concentration
- Prepares for meditation

Yoga breathing exercises, called pranayama, can be done at the beginning of each yoga session, at the end or by themselves. There are multiple benefits. *Prana* in Sanskrit is the "vital life force," that which gives us breath and life. Controlling the breath with these exercises is a start to learn how to control the vital life force, that which gives us energy and sustains us. With daily practice the benefits are infinite, including bringing more oxygen to the blood and cells of the body, purifying the nerves and calming the mind. As the yoga master T Krishnamacharya said: "Breath is central to Yoga because breath is central to life...and Yoga is about life."

Pranayama

To begin, lie down on the floor, with the back on the ground, sitting tall, cross-legged on the floor or in a chair. If you are sitting in a chair, have the feet hip-width apart, with the feet on the floor. (If you are in wheelchair, modify as needed.) Sit tall for Alternate Nostril Breath. Slow Deep Breathing and Three-Part Breath (Full Yogic Breath) can also be done lying down if needed (see the photos on the following pages). Sitting upright creates a feeling of centering the mind and creating alertness. At the end of the yoga exercises, or

Yoga for Everyone!

before relaxation, this can be done in a relaxation pose or lying down for relaxation effects.

Precautions: Take slow, deep breaths if the breathing techniques cause you discomfort or dizziness. Stop the exercise and rest. Try it again when you are ready. Only continue if you are comfortable and feel at ease. All of the breathing exercises in this book are safe for prenatal yoga (all trimesters).

Slow Deep Breathing

Sit tall with your eyes closed. You can also do this from any of the relaxation yoga poses in this book, including Legs Up On the Chair Pose and Relaxation Pose.

Take slow, deep, rhythmic breaths. Inhale and exhale through the nose (if able). Inhale for 3 counts. Exhale for 3 counts. While you count, you can mentally add an "*Aum* (OM)" mantra in between the numbers. (Ex: Om 1, Om 2, etc.) There should be no strain. The shoulders, face and throat remain relaxed. If comfortable, you can increase the breath to 4 counts as you inhale, and 4 counts as you exhale.

This breath type can be done during all yoga postures *(asanas)* too. This is good to do throughout the day, anywhere or anytime, especially in moments when you feel overwhelmed, anxious, angry or stressed out. Be aware of the breath as it connects to the body. Soon your emotions and mind will follow the breath for a deep sense of calm and inner peace.

Benefits: Centers the mind, reduces anxiety, stimulates the parasympathetic nervous system for calming, helps regulate sleep and digestive imbalances. This is a simple and effective 'yogic tool' that can be done anywhere without anyone even knowing you are practicing yoga!

Full Yogic Breath (Three-Part Breath)

Sit tall (either cross-legged on the floor, or in a chair). Bring one hand to the navel area (belly) and the other hand to the upper chest, as in the photo on the following page. Inhale into the belly (push your hands out with the belly as you inhale, expanding the lower belly like a balloon, with no strain.) Exhale and relax. Inhale and exhale for 3 counts each. Inhale into the lower abdomen, then the middle torso, then the upper chest in 3 parts. Exhale in reverse, in 3 counts. When you feel comfortable with the breath, you can relax the hands on the thighs and continue. Repeat 3-10 rounds. Note: You can mentally repeat, "OM 1, OM 2, OM 3", as you count, adding the mantra OM between each number.

Photo: Hands on Abdomen for Full Yogic Breath

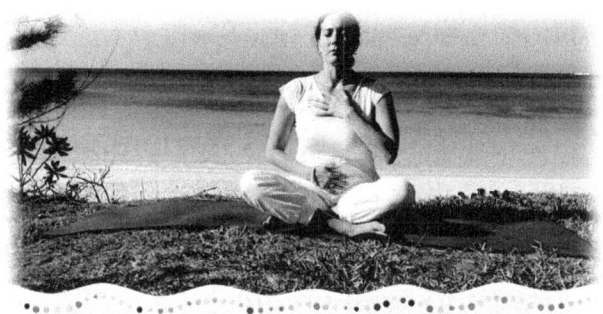

Sukhasana (Easy Pose), Full Yogi Breath

Benefits: Relaxes the stomach, calms and centers the mind, stimulates the parasympathetic nervous system. You can do this anywhere.

Three-Part Breath Lying Down

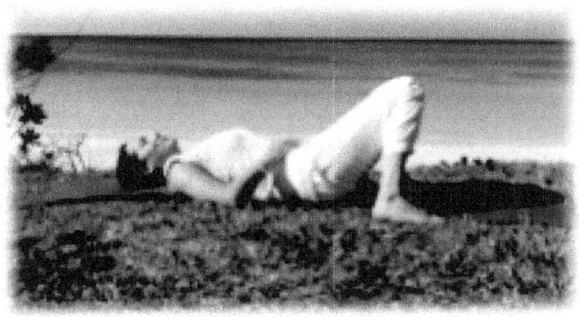

Alternate Nostril Breath

Sitting in a cross-legged seat, or sitting tall in chair, place the right hand in *Vishnu Mudra* (index and, alternating sides. If you are more comfortable or as needed, you can do this with the palm flat and the fingers stretched up. Switch from the index middle finger in towards the palm). See the photos on the following pages. Use the thumb to close the right nostril and the ring finger to close the left nostril finger to close the left nostril and the ring finger to close the right nostril.

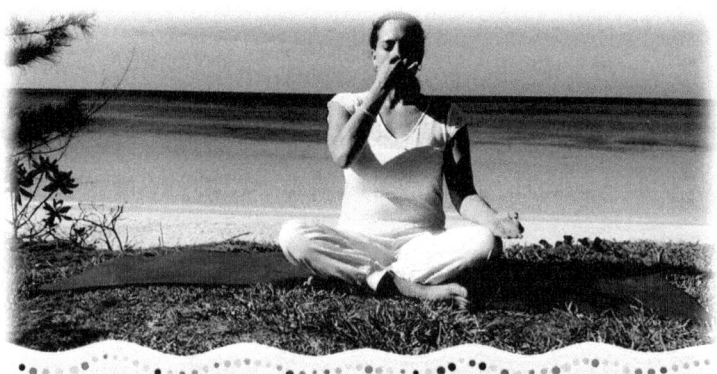

Pranayama: Alternate Nostril Breath

Inhale through the left nostril for 4 counts (block the right nostril with the thumb). Exhale through the right nostril for 8 counts, using the hand position above to close and release the alternating nostrils. Inhale through the right nostril for 4 counts and exhale through the left nostril for

8 counts. Repeat 3 to 12 rounds. The focus is on the third eye (between the eyebrows), with the eyes closed during this exercise. Keep the spine tall yet relaxed.

Return to slow, deep breathing at any point and rest the arm if needed. *Pranayama* works best when the body is relaxed.

Photos below (left): Palm Flat Adaption

Photo below (right): *Vishnu Mudra*

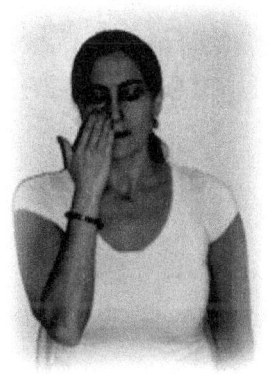 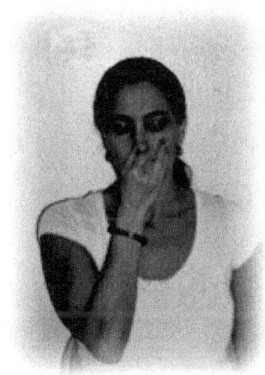

Benefits: Balances the right and left-brain and the energies of the body, calms for the nervous system and mind, improves sleep and concentration abilities, regulates the digestive functions by stimulating the relaxation response and turns the focus inward. This is also a useful preparation for meditation.

"But when the breath is calmed the mind too will be still, and the yogi achieves long life. Therefore, one should learn to control the breath." ~Svatmarama, Hatha Yoga Pradipika

"For breath is life, and if you breathe well you will live long on earth." ~Sanskrit Proverb

"Feelings come and go like clouds in a windy sky. Conscious breathing is my anchor." ~Thích Nhất Hạnh

Meditation

10

In Chapter 10, Meditation

Meditation Benefits
- Brings clarity
- Inspires creativity
- Increases well-being
- Improves concentration
- Brings deep inner peace

Selected Yoga Sutras (from Patanjali)

Sutra 1.2 (Sanskrit):
yogascittavrittinirodhah

Translation: Yoga is the ability to focus the mind towards one point or object and sustain focus in that direction without distraction. Or, Yoga is the stopping of the mind fluctuations.

Sutra 1.14 (Sanskrit) *sa tu dirghakala nairantarya satkara asevitah drdhabhumih*

Translation: Consistent, alert practice with enthusiasm is the firm foundation for stopping the mind fluctuations.

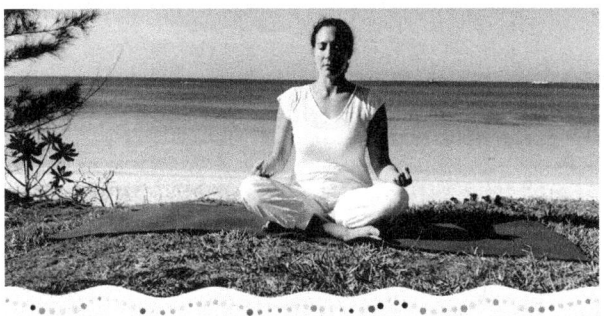
Meditation: Breathe. Observe.

Meditation

Meditation is a time-tested tool for stress reduction and increasing inner peace. It is calming for the mind, brings clarity and increases intuition and our ability to concentrate. In Sanskrit, meditation or *dhyana* is the ability to hold the focus of the mind on one object without distraction until you are absorbed in the focal point, merging with that point of focus. Focusing on a candle (*tratak*, or "eye gazing"), a sound, or mantra or breath are some common focal points. Try to pick something calming or uplifting for the mind.

You can gain many health benefits. For instance, meditation has been studied and proven to reduce heart disease. However, studying it alone does not give you the full benefit. It only works when you do it!

Thinking of meditation, intending to practice

and learning its philosophy are helpful but alone will not give you the fruits of the practice. When meditation is done with consistent practice, regardless of how busy the mind is, we can access a deep well of joy and peace. Often my yoga students say that they or their minds need to meditate. When we sit still, regardless of the reasons why we think we can't, that act of discipline teaches us again and again that we are the masters of our own minds and more than our thoughts alone. Who is the silent witness and knower of all your thoughts? Let's check it out, in one short but sweet minute.

How to Meditate

Find a quiet place. Sit in a comfortable position with your spine tall but not tense. In a chair, you can sit tall with the feet on the floor. Support the lower back with a pillow if needed. Close your eyes. Bring yourself into the present moment. Become aware of your body and its surroundings. Take a few deep sighs. Inhale through the nose. Exhale through the mouth or nose. Start to regulate the breath. Begin slow, rhythmic, deep breathing. Start to observe the breath. Allow the mind to wander at first. It may jump around, but will eventually become quiet. Focus on a point between the eyebrows or the heart area where the mind can rest. When the mind drifts, bring it back to the moment and become aware of the breath. Start with one minute a day. Increase the meditation period gradually over time. Practice, practice, practice!

Be patient with yourself. This takes time to develop. However, the benefits are worth it! If you meditate daily, you will be able to face life with more peace and inner strength, having an anchor within yourself through difficult times. Even if the mind does not seem calm and thoughts are endless, you can still receive the Benefits: and feel more centered throughout your day. Consistent practice is key.

"Get up now. This is Brahmamuhurta (Auspicious Early Morning Time). Everywhere is silence. Nature herself is at peace. Now you can retire peacefully into the inner chambers of your heart."Sivananda

"By cleansing your mind your soul will shine through you." Yogi Bhajan

"The art of meditation is very simple: to clean your mind. The wheel of life has two sides to it, body and mind. And soul is the axle on which it goes on and on. We meditate because we want a clear mind. A clear mind can give you intuition and intuition can let you know the cause and effects. For the effects you don't want to face, you drop the cause. You can't drop the effect." Yogi Bhajan

"Regular meditation opens the avenues of intuitional knowledge, makes the mind calm and steady, awakens an ecstatic feeling, and brings the practitioner in contact with the source of his/her very being." Sivananda

"The soul loves to meditate, for in contact with the Spirit lies its greatest joy. If, then, you experience mental resistance during meditation, remember that reluctance to meditate comes from the ego; it doesn't belong to the soul."
Paramhansa Yogananda

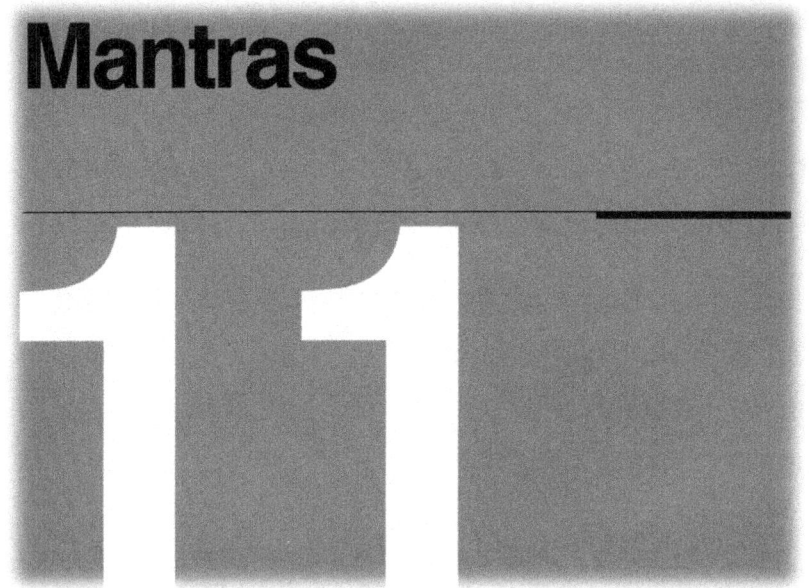

Mantras

11

In Chapter 11, Mantras

Benefits of Mantras
- Brings joy
- Calms the mind
- Increases harmony
- Improves concentration
- Gives one-pointed focus
- Balances the chakras
- Improves memory
  - Kirtan Kriya for clarity

"Mantra Yoga is an exact science. 'Mananat Trayate Iti Mantrah-by the Manan (constant thinking or recollection) of which one is released from the round of births and deaths is Mantra.'

Every Mantra has a Rishi who gave it to the world; a Matra, a Devata, the Bija or seed which gives it a special power, the Sakti and the Kilakam or the pillar.

A Mantra is divinity. Mantra and its presiding Devata are one. The Mantra itself is Devata. Mantra is divine power, Daivi Sakti, manifesting in a sound body. Constant repetition of the Mantra with faith, devotion and purity augments the Sakti or power of the aspirant, purifies and awakens the Mantra Chaitanya latent in the Mantra and bestows on the Sadhaka, Mantra Siddhi, illumination, freedom, peace, eternal bliss, immortality." Swami Sivananda

Yoga is commonly thought of as physical exercises and breathing techniques, perhaps with some relaxation. However, that is part of Hatha Yoga. There are also other branches of yoga that do not require any physical abilities or mobility.

The Sivananda Yoga lineage summarizes the paths of yoga in this way: "There are four main

paths of Yoga - Karma Yoga, Bhakti Yoga, Raja Yoga and Jnana Yoga. Each is suited to a different temperament or approach to life…. Swami Sivananda recognized that every Yogi, or human being for that matter, possesses and identifies with each of these elements: Intellect, heart, body and mind. He therefore advocated that everyone practice certain techniques from each path. This came to be known as the Yoga of Synthesis. He also taught that, in accordance with individual temperament and taste, one can emphasize the practice of certain Yogas over others."
www.sivananda.org

Mantras and chanting are apart of Bhakti Yoga, which is the yogic path of devotion. This can be done at the end of the yoga session or on its own. Feel the joy in your heart and soul and you chant and sing with devotion. Chanting is not like singing or performing. Your voice does not have to be "good" or you do not have to feel it is "good" to chant and feel the inner joy it brings. If you are new to chanting and prefer to chant silently, you can still feel and reap the benefits. Although you can chant in any language, the Sanskrit language is said to have a spiritual resonance, as it was spoken from the gurus from thousands of years ago and carried through the ages.

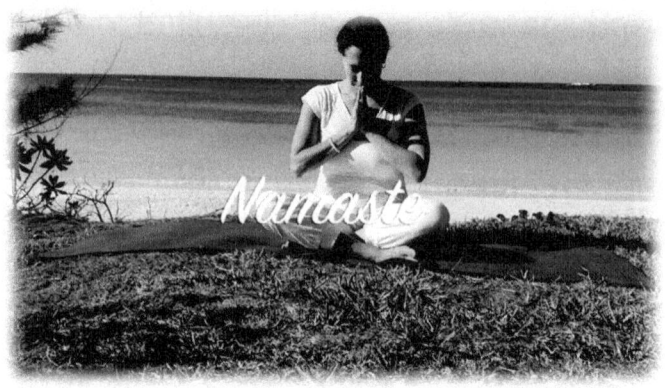

Namaste is often thought of as a mantra. In fact it is a greeting, for hello and goodbye as used often in India and Nepal. It means "the divine or truth in me, honors the divine or truth in you."

Mantras

AUM (OM)

Inhale. As you exhale, chant *AUM* (OM). Feel as if you are chanting from deep within the navel center, letting the sound current (wave) rise up to the third eye point (point between the eyebrows). Imagine that every cell of your body is being healed by the sacred primordial sound of the universe: *AUM*.

Universal prayer for all beings:

Lokha, Samasta Sukino, Bhavantu (Repeat 3x)

Aum Shanti, Shanti, Shanti-e

Translation: May all beings in all worlds be happy and free. Peace in our bodies, Peace in our minds, Peace to all souls.

Ancient prayer for knowing our true Self:

Asato Ma Sat Gamaya

Tamasoma Jyotir Gamaya

Mrityor Maamritam Gamaya

Aum Shanti, Shanti, Shanti-e

Lead us from the unreal to the real.

Lead us from darkness to light.

Lead us from fear of death/anxiety,

To knowledge of our soul's immortality.

Om Peace, Peace, Peace.

Kirtan Kriya for Memory Improvement

Yogi Bhajan, who brought Kundalini Yoga to the west, taught Kirtan Kriya. It is a combination of mantras and mudras (chants and hand postures). The mantras are from the Gurmukhi script from India. The other chants in the book and the names of the yoga postures are in the Sanskrit language, also from India.

The following description of how to do this exercise (or meditation) is written by the Alzheimer's Research & Prevention Foundation. (Visit www.alzheimersprevention.org for more details on how their evidence-based study showed that this Kirtan Kriya improved memory in patients suffering from mild cognitive impairment (MCI) and early Alzheimer's.)

The Alzheimer's Research & Prevention Foundation has assembled this information on the Kirtan Kriya singing exercise for medical professionals, the public, caregivers, the media and anyone interested in improving brain function and slowing memory loss.

The Kirtan Kriya exercise uses the primal

sounds and is meant to be practiced for greater attention, concentration, focus, improved short-term memory and better mood. The primal sounds consist of: Saa – means Birth or Infinity, Taa – means Life, Naa – means Death or Transformation, Maa – means Rebirth.

The sounds are chanted repeatedly and in order (i.e., Saa Taa Naa Maa). You can start with 3 minutes until you are familiar with the technique, using the time ratio of 30 s:30 s:60 s:30 s:30 s and then building up to a full 12 minutes.

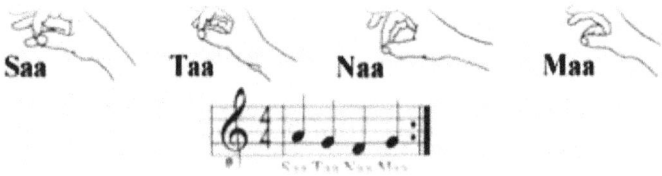

Photo below: L Form Visualization

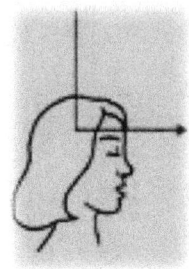

Chakra Balance Chant

Chakra in Sanskrit means "wheel". It is a vortex of energy, according to Indian philosophy, believed to be located along the central channel of the body. There are 7 *chakras*. Bring attention to each *chakra* and chant the associated mantra 3-8x as you keep the focus on the energy center. You can chant out loud or silently. You can also visualize the color associated with each *chakra*. These are seed *(bija)* mantras. *See the next page.*

- LAM- 1st chakra (root)

- VAM- 2nd chakra (sacral/navel)

- RAM- 3rd chakra (solar plexus)

- YAM- 4th chakra (heart)

- HAM"- 5th chakra (throat)

- AUM - 6th chakra (third eye/brow point)

- OM/silence- 7th chakra (crown)

Benefits: Improves concentration, calms the mind and nervous system, balances the energy of the body, turns the mental focus inward, prepares the mind for meditation.

Chakra Balance Chant *(Bija Mantras)*

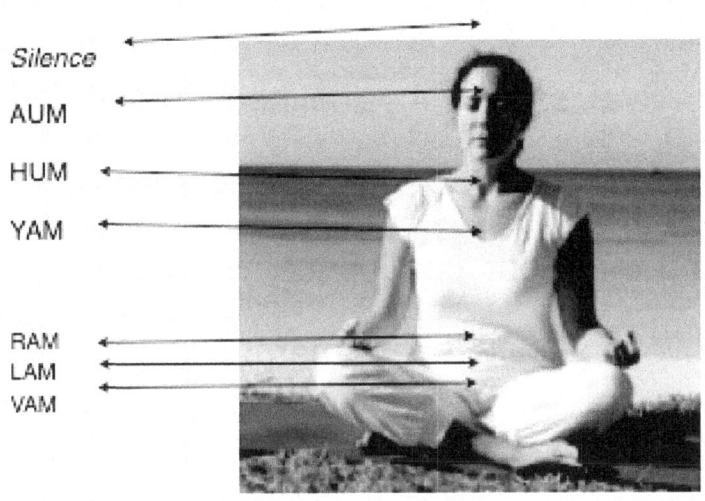

Silence

AUM

HUM

YAM

RAM
LAM
VAM

Colors associated with 7 Chakras

1st (base of spine) Red

2nd (sacral area/reproductive organs) Orange

3rd (abdomen, between naval & spine) Yellow

4th (heart center) Green

5th (throat center) Light Blue

6th (slightly above center of eyebrows) Indigo

7th (2" above top of the head) White or Violet

7 Chakras Relations

1st -Survival, safety, physical body, grounding

2nd -Creative energy, sexuality, pleasure

3rd -Empowerment, confidence, will power

4th -Love, self-love, heart energy, emotions

5th -Communication, truth, expressing truth

6th -Intuition, clarity, meditation, insight

7th -Spiritual and physical connection, oneness

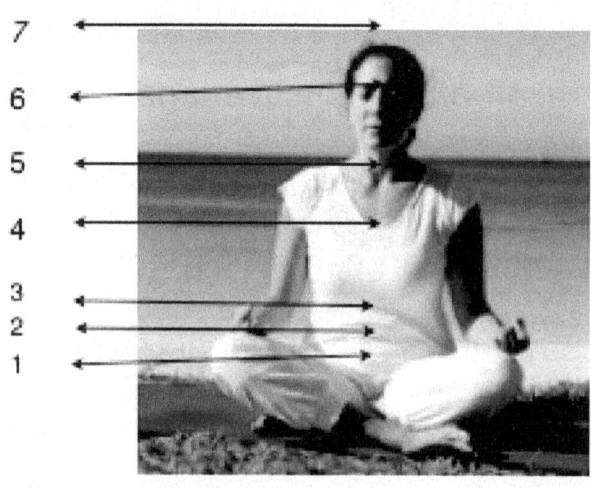

About the Author

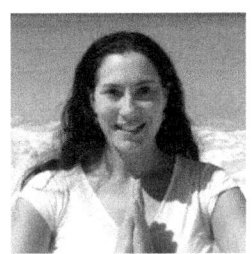

Stacie Dooreck was born and raised a vegetarian and taken to yoga ashrams since birth. Stacie began teaching yoga in 1995 (Sivananda Yoga Certified) and since became certified to teach prenatal yoga, Gentle Integral Yoga and Kundalini Yoga as taught by Yogi Bhajan. In addition, Stacie trained at the advanced studies program at the Iyengar Institute of San Francisco and continued to study with the yoga masters.

After needing to adapt her own yoga practice during an illness and receiving its healing benefits, Stacie loves to share the joy of yoga with others. Stacie created and leads the **SunLight Chair Yoga** teacher trainings and wrote SunLight Chair Yoga: yoga for everyone! books (two editions and an ebook).

Stacie has been featured on KQED/NPR radio, CBS Healthwatch news, Albuquerque News, Albuquerque Journal, San Francisco Yoga

Magazine, LA Yoga Magazine, Marin Magazine and many others.

"Stacie is breathing new life in South Florida seniors." -CBS Heathwatch Miami News 2014

"Stacie's work of the heart is helping others to feel sunshine amid the challenges of human life at every stage of being. The world needs more sunshine yoga teachers like Stacie." San Francisco Yoga Magazine 2017

Stacie also writes for various publications and a monthly Yogatips eletter.

On www.sunlightchairyoga.com you can watch videos and audio links to:

- Learn the Chair Yoga Sun Salutations

- Learn Chair Yoga flow sequences

- View a Chair Yoga demo at Bahamas Ashram

- Learn Alternate Nostril Breathing for Calming

- Listen to Inquire Within Podcast on Chair Yoga

- Listen to Chair Yoga for Caregivers on Alzheimer's Speaks Radio & Chair Yoga with Stacie on Body Wisdom with Dr. Mich ele

Also Available:

3 DVDs: Chair Yoga, Gentle Yoga, Hatha Yoga

SunLight Yoga Publishers:

Email: info@sunlightyoga.com

Facebook: www.facebook.com/yogainchairs

Twitter: www.twitter/yogainchairs

Website: www.sunlightchairyoga.com

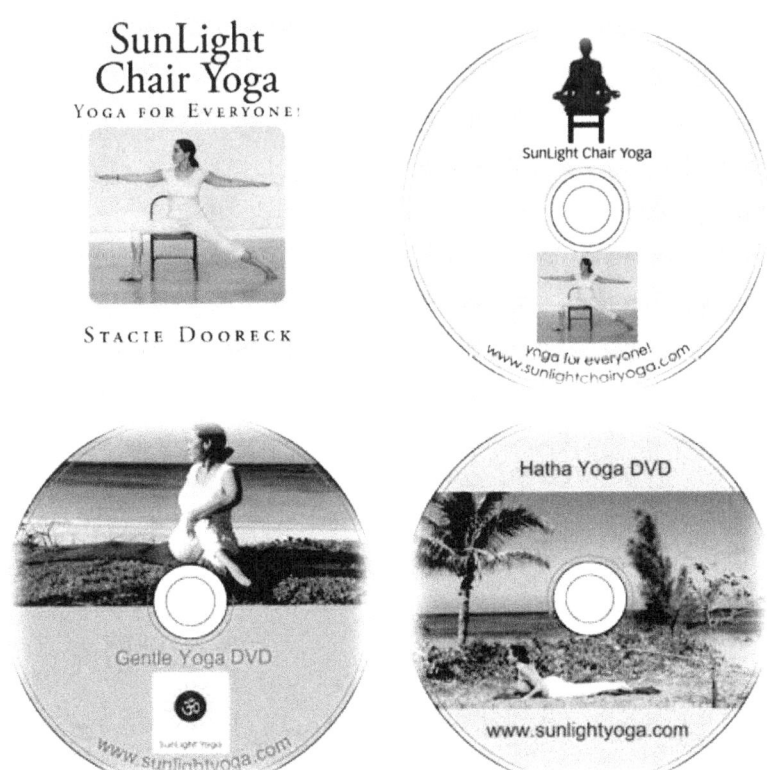

88807285R00202

Made in the USA
Columbia, SC
10 February 2018